STAND TALLER ~ LIVE LONGER

Copyright 2008 © All rights reserved. Steven P. Weiniger DC

Library of Congress Cataloging-in-Publication Data available on Request

ISBN-13 - 978-0-9797136-0-6
ISBN-10 - 0-9797136-0-9

Published by BodyZone LLC
3000 Old Alabama Road
Suite 119-352
Alpharetta, Georgia USA 30022
770-922-0700
www.standtallerlivelonger.com

Photography
Eric Bern Studio
Ed Wolkis Photography
John Ramspott

Editing
George Weinstein

Models
Dr. Craig Aaron
Kate Harbin
Molly Harbin
Alex Nesbit
Renee North
Aubrey Steinbaum
Erica Weiniger
Lauren Weiniger
Renee Weiniger
Amy Wolkis

Book design
Cecilia Sorochin & Yanina Arabena for Sorodesign
Typeset
DIN Regular 9pt combined with Adobe Garamond Pro Italic

Trademarks
BodyZone.com, the BodyZone.com logo, Move, Feel and Be Well, and StrongPosture and related trade dress are trademarks or registered trademarks of BodyZone LLC or Steven P. Weiniger D.C. and may not be used without prior written permission.

Limits of Liability
The intention of this book is solely informational and educational. The exercises, techniques and advice contained herein are meant to supplement, and not to be a substitute for, the advice of a professional, and should not be used to treat a serious ailment without prior consultation with a qualified health care professional. In particular, your physician needs to know if you have heart trouble, high blood pressure, arthritis, if you often feel dizzy or have chest pains, or if you have any other significant health problem or concern.

STAND TALLER ~ LIVE LONGER

AN ANTI-AGING STRATEGY

10 Minutes a Day to Keep Your Body Active and Pain-Free

by Steven P. Weiniger DC

This book is dedicated to my mom,
Lucille Sheier Friedman Weiniger,
for teaching me to balance the perspectives of expecting
to live forever while embracing each day

and to my dad, Julius Weiniger,
for teaching me to work hard for dreams

Acknowledgments

Many thanks to Ed Wolkis and Eric Bern, for your invaluable
friendship, time and ideas.

Thank you Dr. Allen Weiniger and Dr. Bruce Miron for your
insights and feedback as the book developed.

Thanks to Dr. Craig Aaron, a great model and an excellent
doctor.

Thank you, George Weinstein, for your advice and reading,
and reading and
re-reading.

Thank you Jeff, Ceci, Yanina and others at Sorodesign for
your patience with endless revisions.

Thanks also to my family, friends and colleagues - I am
very appreciative for your suggestions, help and contributions to this effort.

And to the kids, Lauren, Erica and Alex, thanks for never
getting tired of hearing about posture!

With gratitude and love to my wife, partner, muse and coach, Renée,
for her invaluable contributions and wisdom in this book and along the path of life

TABLE OF **CONTENTS**

21

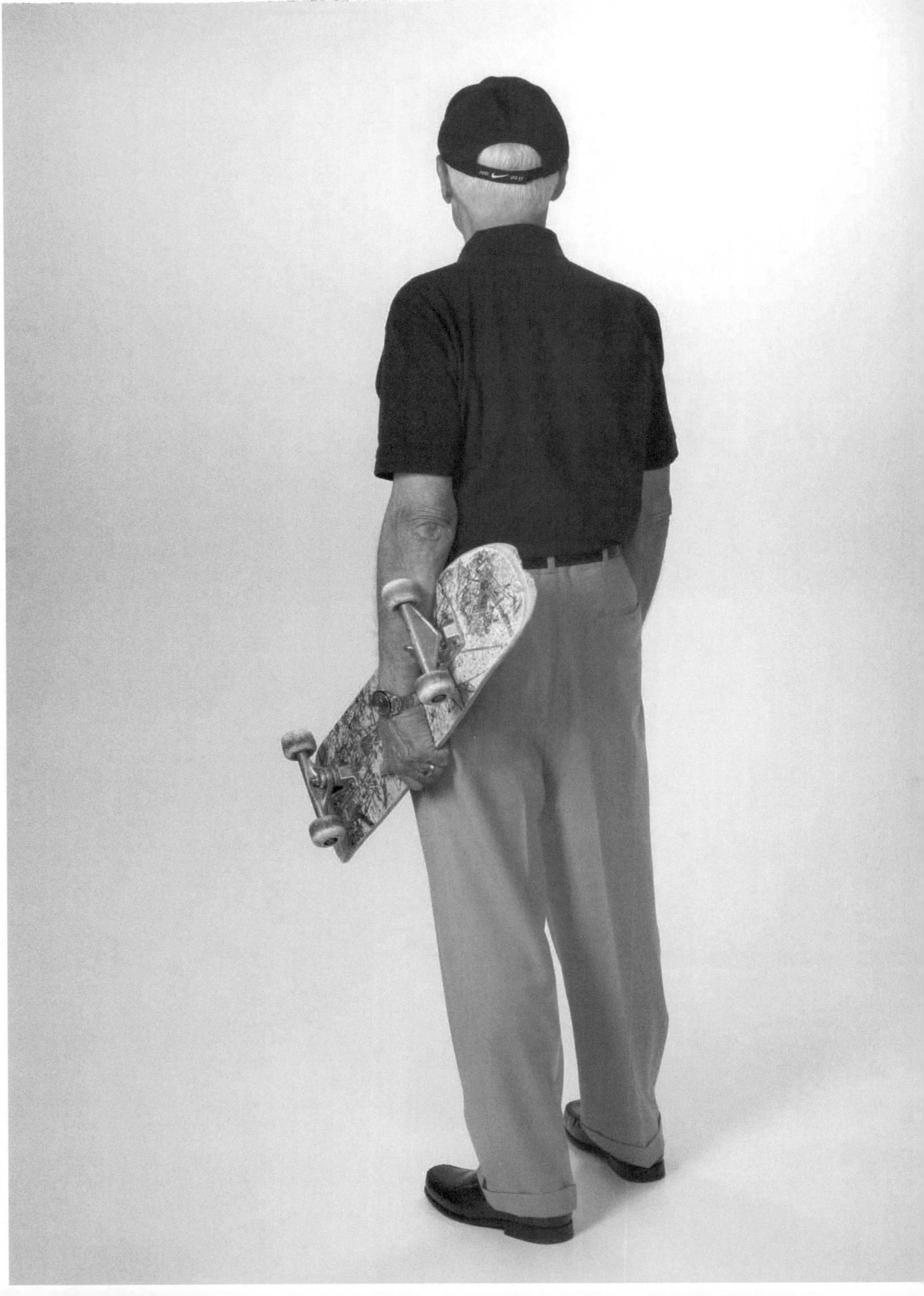

1 Posture, Pain and Aging

The path to poor posture, and the way back again

"He's in great shape. That's how I want to be at his age."

Figure 1-1a How old does this man look?

Have you ever seen a man from behind and thought he was your father's age, and then were surprised to see the face of someone younger than you? Or, have you ever seen a woman from behind and thought she was your age, and then were surprised to see she was old enough to be your grandmother?

Standing in line at the supermarket, walking in the park, waiting at the airport, or wherever I people-watch, I frequently see someone whose posture and motion defies their age. It might be the bent-over man whose posture reminds me of my grandfather, but whose face is closer in age to my own. Or I might see a woman with a toddler, and only on overhearing their conversation do I realize she is the child's grandmother. If you have noticed the same thing, have you ever wondered why some lucky people in their seventies, eighties, or even nineties move and look young. Is it their skin? Or is it how they move and carry themselves? In other words, is it their posture?

4| Not only does language reflect the link between posture, personality, and emotion, but clinically observing posture and assessing how someone moves can be a window into looking at their general health.

The relationship between posture and general health is not surprising since posture is the physical end result of how your body deals with the millions of inputs about your environment that the brain receives from the nervous system every second. In fact, if you want to know how a person is feeling today, look at their posture and how they move. Is their motion stiff and guarded, like an old person? Or do they move smoothly, with grace and ease? When someone has StrongPosture™, you look at them and know they have energy and vitality.

My goal in writing this book is to teach you about your body, and provide a blueprint to first become conscious of posture, and then integrate StrongPosture™ exercises into your daily routine to literally change how you move. Conscious StrongPosture™ exercises can help keep your body moving as it was designed to and slow, and even reverse, the degeneration of posture with age.

This book will present some ideas that may challenge your preconceptions, and others may give you what I call an "AH-HA moment." An AH-HA moment is when something clicks in your mind, and suddenly you "get it." Most people are kinesthetic learners, and learn best when they can feel and touch something to truly understand it. Many concepts are accompanied by TRY THIS demonstrations, which kinesthetically demonstrate how your body moves. If a picture is worth a thousand words, feeling something is worth a thousand pictures.

*Posture Is **How** You Balance Your Body*

Did you ever notice that images you see in books or posters teaching good posture, whether it's how to "stand straight" or sit at your computer in an "ergonomically correct" position, are almost always drawings and not photographs? The reason is that "ideal" posture is just that...an ideal. Real people don't have "perfect posture" because no one is perfect. Our posture is how our bodies have adapted to the life we are living.

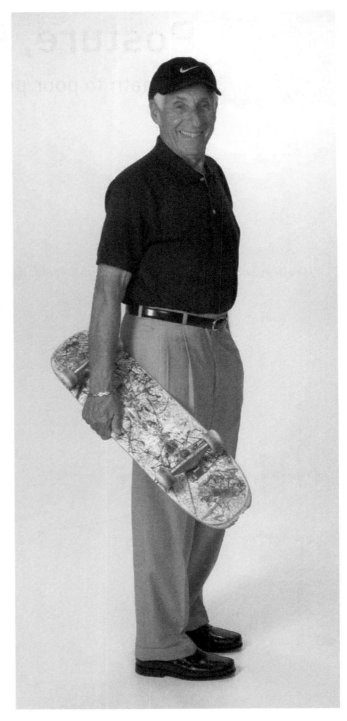

▲ **Figure 1-1b** Strong Posture is why this 80 year old man looks...and feels...younger than his years.

Wrong vs. StrongPosture™

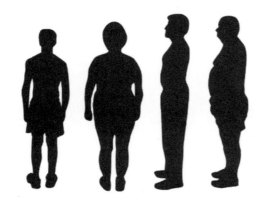

▲ **Figure 1-2** Who has balanced posture?

- **Q:** *Which of these postures is balanced?*

  A: All of them!

Anyone who is standing up is, by definition, balanced, but how well are they balanced is a different question. Posture is the practical end result of how you balance your body. Posture is dynamic, not static, and is a trade off between flexibility and stability, between motion and effort. Postural balance is the ability to control your body's position in space, and keep your body upright and stable, especially when challenged. Poorly balanced posture requires more energy to stay upright, causing some areas to carry more stress and wear out more quickly than nature intended.

There is no one "perfect" posture.

Posture is about more than standing straight, and improving posture involves more than just telling someone to stand straight and keep their shoulders back. Improving posture means strengthening how the body balances, and how it moves.

Though there is no one perfect posture, there are better and worse postures. Posture is not just how you stand, but it's also how you balance your body when you sit. We live in a sitting society. Sitting is the 21st century posture, and our couch potato lifehabits are a primary cause of the epidemic of back pain and other motion-based problems afflicting our society.

In our technological lifestyle, people sit A LOT, spending more than half their waking lives folded in a cramped sitting position. When:

- **Driving:** In 2001 Americans spent an average of 62 minutes a day driving, up from 49 minutes a day in 1990, an extra 80 hours each year spent sitting slouched in poor posture. Not only does looking straight ahead, hands on wheel, stress the body by locking us in a fixed position, but sitting up and fighting the constant engine and road vibration is an often unrecognized factor in many back pain problems[i].

- **Working:** For 75% of us, this is sedentary labor such as sitting at a desk hunched over in front of a computer.

- **Relaxing:** Sitting down to eat or watch TV, surfing the web or playing videogames.

Many people with back problems say they have poor posture. They are usually right. Experts all agree that mechanically related back problems are a large and growing health and economic problem for modern society. Whether you look at low back, middle back, or neck pain, there is no argument that the costs are enormous[ii]. A 2004 **Newsweek** cover story reported that back pain costs America $100 billion a year in medical bills, disability, and lost productivity!

The human body is designed to walk and run, not sit. When we stand erect we can use our eyes to see ahead, walk upright, and use our hands to wave at a friend, throw a rock, or gather berries. To stand erect, we must balance the three postural weight centers of the human frame: the head, the chest, and the pelvis. The problem begins when we work the deep core muscles balancing our body in only a small part of their full range of motion-- muscles adapt and atrophy, and over time the characteristic slump of old age develops.

Now, this is not to say that everyone has poor posture. But if you spend a big chunk of your life sitting, unless you are actively doing something to counteract your habits, your posture will suffer. You are what you do, and contrary to popular belief, practice doesn't make perfect.
The truth is, **practice makes permanent**.

61

»TRY THIS: *Balancing Act*
Why poor posture causes fatigue and stress.

- Take a broom, a golf club, or anything long with a handle, grasp the end of the handle and balance it upside down in one hand.

- Hold the broom straight up in the air.

> **Notice:** It is easy when you keep it upright and balanced
> Now, let the broom lean over a foot or so to one side.
> It gets a LOT heavier, because you must work harder to hold up the object.
>
> Like the club or broom, your body has to balance, and it's harder to balance a misaligned body. And as we will see, your posture is quite literally how you balance your body.

Many patients tell me this demonstration really helped them realize how poor body mechanics creates fatigue and stress. Just as you need to work harder to support the broom, poor balance takes more energy. Your sense of balance determines your posture, so when someone stands with a distorted posture, they are not symmetrical, and they will unconsciously work muscles harder to compensate and maintain balance. After all, if they don't maintain balance, they fall down.

> I use this demonstration to answer the patients who ask me, "Why do I feel lighter after an adjustment?" I explain that the broom off-balance is you before an adjustment; the aligned broom is you after an adjustment. When adjusted and aligned, joints move symmetrically and in harmony with the rest of the body so biomechanically speaking, you balance more effectively and your body moves more efficiently.

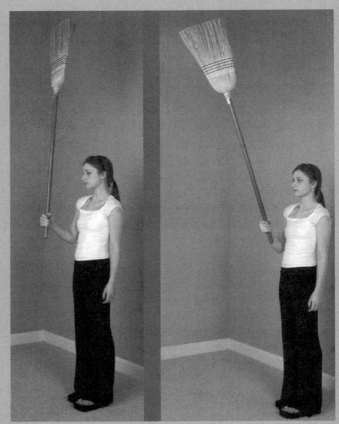

▲ **Figure 1-3** Balancing a broom (or golf club) vertically takes less effort

▲ **Figure 1-4** The greater deviation from vertical, the greater the effort to keep it balanced

Posture and Habits

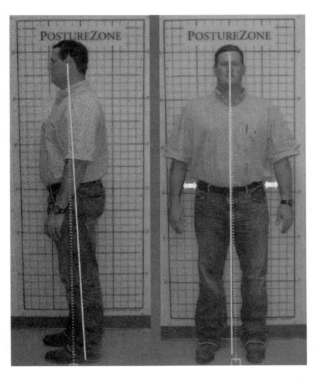

 Figure 1-5 Posture symmetry

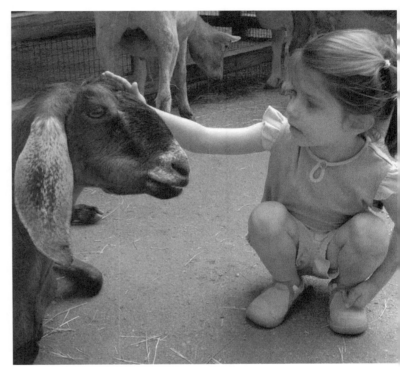

▲ **Figure 1-6** Child squatting with feet flat and grounded

Ideal posture is symmetrical and equally proportioned from left to right. However, most people do not have ideal bodies. Posture pictures of practically every patient I see show a high shoulder, a low hip, or loss of the normal forward curve in their neck. People adapt to their injury and habits, and so their body motion also adapts.

The bent-over posture of a 60-year-old woman with a dowager's hump has its seeds in the posture of a 16-year-old girl slumping in front of the TV for hours on end. Also, poor adaptive posture habits usually worsen with age, causing chronic problems such as neck and back pain, stress and chronic fatigue.

Different motions cause different muscles to strengthen and others to weaken with neglect. Our body changes with our habits. For example, a child can squat comfortably, heels on the ground, and play or eat for an extended period of time. In primitive aboriginal cultures, adult women even give birth in a squatting position. And while a dancer with good posture

may be able to keep both her heels on the ground when squatting, the deconditioned computer user of 35 (and most other modern adults) usually cannot come anywhere near squatting without lifting their heels, a sure sign of adaptively tight leg muscles.

Our habits are what we do, and they shape our posture. There is a saying, "The more you sit, the lazier you get." It is also true that the more you sit, the tighter you get. It is not surprising that studies show half of all computer workers report suffering pain[iii].

Poor posture usually gets progressively worse with age, ultimately making slouchers look, and feel, far older than they should.

> "Some low back pain is caused and all low back pain *is aggravated by poor sitting posture.*"
> Robin McKenzie, noted back pain expert

81

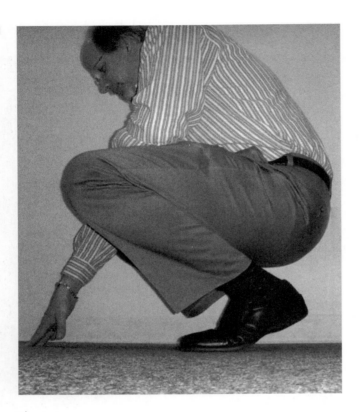

▲ **Figure 1-7** Adult squatting with heels lifted

Improving posture means strengthening how you balance your body, and reducing mechanical stress on your body. Like balancing a broom at a 45° angle, poor posture stresses muscles and joints to make you look and feel old because it is biomechanically ineffective.

StrongPosture™ comes from the deep, core muscles of the body. As the name implies, the core muscles are the innermost muscles connecting and stabilizing the torso over the pelvis. We stabilize without thinking as we stand on two legs and constantly balance our head over our torso, and our torso over our pelvis. As we will see, our posture is literally how the spine—a flexible rod—and our muscles constantly work, compensate, and adapt to keep us upright.

Posture, Pain, and Living Long

Everyone knows people lose height as they age, but did you know your life can get shorter as you get shorter? According to a recent 20-year study, there is a strong correlation between losing height and mortality[iv]. Researchers at the University of London divided 4,200 men aged 40-59 into 4 groups by how much height they lost over 20 years.

> Less than 1 cm
> 1-2 cm
> 2-3 cm
> Over 3 cm

Men who lost over 3 cm of height had 1.45 times the risk of dying as compared to those losing less than 1 cm. The authors speculated that the physical restriction of the lungs and abdominal organs caused significantly greater risk of cardiovascular disease, stroke and respiratory mortality. In other words,

Stand Taller and Live Longer

In addition, as the unbalanced biomechanical stress of asymmetric posture not only molds muscles and ligaments, but over time the bones themselves actually bend and collapse[v].

> Osteoporosis, a loss of bone calcium common in post-menopausal women, is commonly pointed to as a cause of compression fractures and the "dowager's hump" posture, leading to loss of height. However, the Harvard Medical School Adviser[vi] recently asserted that despite the bone-weakening effects of osteoporosis:
> "Some research suggests that vertebral fractures have been overrated as a cause of height loss and hunching. Another big reason may simply be bad posture."

Despite strong evidence that posture exercise helps prevent stooped posture and strengthen balance to prevent falls and fractures[vii], there is little media focus on strengthening posture.

The posture and balance problems associated with aging are commonly accepted as "part of getting old" and therefore are not treated. This is not necessarily true. Unlike the ads for osteoporosis drugs paid for by drug companies, there are no advertising campaigns promoting the significant improvements in posture[viii] and reduction of fractures in post-menopausal women associated with regular StrongPosture™ exercises.

Ironically, another reason to keep your body moving as you advance in years, and why posture-related problems are a growing epidemic in seniors, is that as healthcare improves in other areas people are living longer. The person who suffered a heart attack at age 65 that would have been fatal ten years ago now may live another twenty years, and is at greater risk of posture- and joint-degeneration. The longer people live, the more time the accumulated consequences of postural "sins of their youth" have to catch up with them.

Posture and motion don't only affect how long you live, but also how well you live. Postural and biomechanically related back problems are the number three reason for all doctor visits (the common cold and other respiratory infections are number one and two).

Consider:

- 80 percent of Americans are afflicted with back pain at some point in their lives.
- 65 million Americans suffer from back pain every year.
- Musculoskeletal conditions, including arthritis, low back pain, and repetitive motion strain, are the leading cause of absenteeism[ix], with 2% of the U.S. work force annually suffering a compensable back injury.
- 83% of Americans rely on over-the-counter pain relievers[x].
- 2/3 of the people who have experienced back pain can expect some symptoms every year.
- Low back pain is the most common cause of disability for people under age 45[xi], causing lost productivity in addition to non-monetary costs such as diminished enjoyment of life and the ability to perform normal daily activities.

Young or old, many people with poor posture don't realize they have a problem.

When assessing posture, I am frequently astounded by how many people say they are not in pain, despite displaying significant signs of biomechanical stress. Subtle asymmetries when people stand or walk tell a trained eye, or even a layperson, that someone is uncomfortable.

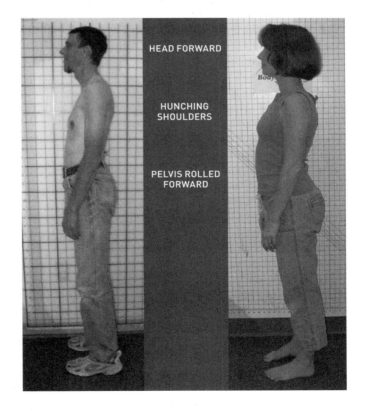

HEAD FORWARD

HUNCHING SHOULDERS

PELVIS ROLLED FORWARD

▲ **Figure 1-8** Everyday adaptive posture

When I question someone with such adaptive postures, they usually admit to either being in "regular" pain, or frequently suffering from some kind of neck, back, joint, muscle, or other postural pain but having learned to medicate or otherwise cope with the problem.

Some people only admit to pain when they can no longer tolerate it, or rationalize their chronic, low-grade discomfort by saying "it just hurts me because I..." and then fill in whatever activity they blame. The computer worker says their neck, or shoulder, or wrists hurt because of working at a keyboard. The salesperson says their feet hurt from standing all day. The forklift operator says their low back hurts from lifting. Such people initially will say they are fine, but when confronted, say they just have "normal pain, but it's OK when I take something for it."

Pain is not normal.

I repeat: Living with pain is not normal. Pain is a sign of tissue damage, stress, injury, breakdown, or other malfunction in the body. In my chiropractic practice, new patients commonly tell me they have "normal" back pain, "normal" wrist pain, and headaches they attribute to "normal" stress. This is insane! Pain is not normal!

Even if you can keep on going, living with pain does not make you a good and virtuous person. It makes you a person in pain who is hurting and living with it. Controlling the pain with over-the-counter medications may work for a little while, but long-term dependence on aspirin, Tylenol®, or other analgesics is not good. These drugs are not as innocent as advertised, and stomach, liver, and kidney diseases are but a few of the consequences of their long-term use.

There is a saying, "Once a back problem, always a back problem." On the other hand, most people's attitude toward pain is pretty much "Out of sight, out of mind." The patient who hobbles into my office and then walks out pain-free will gratefully tell me I "fixed" the problem. At that point, I am delighted that my efforts have helped the pain, and possibly even slowed the progress of breakdown. But, especially if the patient has had pain before or has learned to live with low-grade pain, I know there is still an underlying problem.

My premise has always been that patients (actually, people in general) want to know what is wrong, fix it (permanently if possible), and then forget about it. I remember a man I treated who was upset because he was still having shoulder pain four weeks after he began seeing me for chiropractic care. After reviewing his file, I asked him how his neck pain and headaches were doing. He denied having a neck problem until I showed him where, in his own hand, he had written on his initial paperwork that he suffered neck pain and headaches. Once the pain was gone he had forgotten all about it! On reflection, he realized he was doing better, despite the persistence of the shoulder pain. And two weeks later his shoulder pain was doing much better as well.

Ironically, the desire for a permanent solution leads many people suffering biomechanical problems to radical spinal surgery, despite its far-less-than-enviable record. This desire for a quick, permanent fix can lead to permanent post-surgical tissue adhesions and scars, which in turn set the stage for more biomechanical problems and explains why chiropractors and others addressing such soft tissue and fascial issues help many patients suffering from FBSS (Failed Back Surgery Syndrome—yes, there really is such a condition).

A far more intelligent solution for back problems, albeit one that takes a bit of discipline, is changing how you move and use your body—in other words, your posture. Ten minutes a day of StrongPosture™ exercise can help you become "Posture Conscious" and literally retrain how your body moves. Reprogramming your "normal" posture takes a consistent effort initially to create the habit of daily StrongPosture™ exercise. However, investing a few minutes a day and focusing on your Balance, your Alignment, and your Body Motion will make you conscious of your posture and therefore help strengthen your body's bio-mechanics in everything you do.

People with chronic problems or significant tissue damage may require muscle therapy, fascial therapy, spinal manipulation or other professional help to restore long-lost motion to locked links in the biomechanical chain of motion. But once someone begins to improve as motion is restored, professionals from doctors of chiropractic to muscle therapists and from physical therapists to personal trainers teach their patients (or clients) StrongPosture™ exercises to retrain new patterns of motion. And in addition to recommending regular massage or wellness adjustments for ongoing freedom of motion and drug-free pain control, bodywork professionals recommend daily StrongPosture™ exercises to move, feel and be well.

Posture and Aging

Contrary to popular wisdom, aging alone generally does not cause pain[xii]. We think about chronological years when talking about age, or how long ago we were born. However, there are different ways of looking at age. Before reading this book you may never have thought about how much your posture says about your age, how you feel, and even your quality of life. People agree that aging well is the name of the game. While a youthful appearance and good looks are important to many, aging well is not just about how old you look; it's how old you feel today, and what you can expect for tomorrow. There is a strong argument that how well you function today is as important as when you were born.

People think old and stiff rather than old and weak, for good reason. The common bent-over posture of old age occurs as a result of the body adapting to long-term poor posture, which causes biomechanical stress: muscles tighten and the spine and other joints stiffen and breakdown.

Increasingly people are exercising to stay strong and active, a good thing. There are four aspects of fitness that all work together for good health: strength, cardiovascular, flexibility, and proprioception (or balance). However, workouts focused on breaking a sweat and breathing hard, possibly with a bit of stretching thrown in, work only the first three. Despite being widely recognized as essential for fitness, most people neglect posture and balance training in their exercise programs. This is unfortunate because especially as we age, balance deteriorates and injuries result as people fall down. Every year a third of Americans over 65 suffer a fall[xiii], resulting in 1.8 million Emergency Room visits for fall related injuries in 2003 alone, with 460,000 hospitalization and a sobering 13,700 fatalities[xiv].

However, balance and posture training is not just for old people. Elite athletes and weekend warriors alike can significantly improve both performance and the benefits of exercise. Since posture is HOW you balance your body, when your sense of balance is off your body must compensate to stay upright.

As posture becomes progressively more bent forward, muscles are forced to work harder to keep the body balanced. Some muscles tighten while others weaken with worsening muscle imbalance, which explains why low back pain

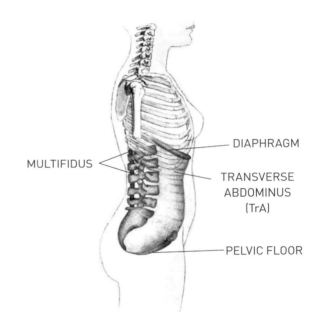

MULTIFIDUS

DIAPHRAGM

TRANSVERSE ABDOMINUS (TrA)

PELVIC FLOOR

Figure 1-9 The deep core muscles essential for StrongPosture™

sufferers show loss of the deep posture control muscles.

> **RESEARCH:** Weaker core muscles correlates with low back pain severity and duration.
> MRIs can measure the cross-section of muscles to assess function and strength. When researchers compared these deep muscles on patients with low back pain for over 12 weeks they found a loss of muscle on the side with pain. The loss of muscle correlated with the severity and the duration of the symptoms: the longer and more severe the pain, the more loss of muscle on the side with pain[xv].

Posture is not just about how you look, but can actually affect how long and how well you live. Research shows that people who move well and have good posture age better. Even small changes in the ability to move has been documented to improve quality of life in older people, and significant

12|

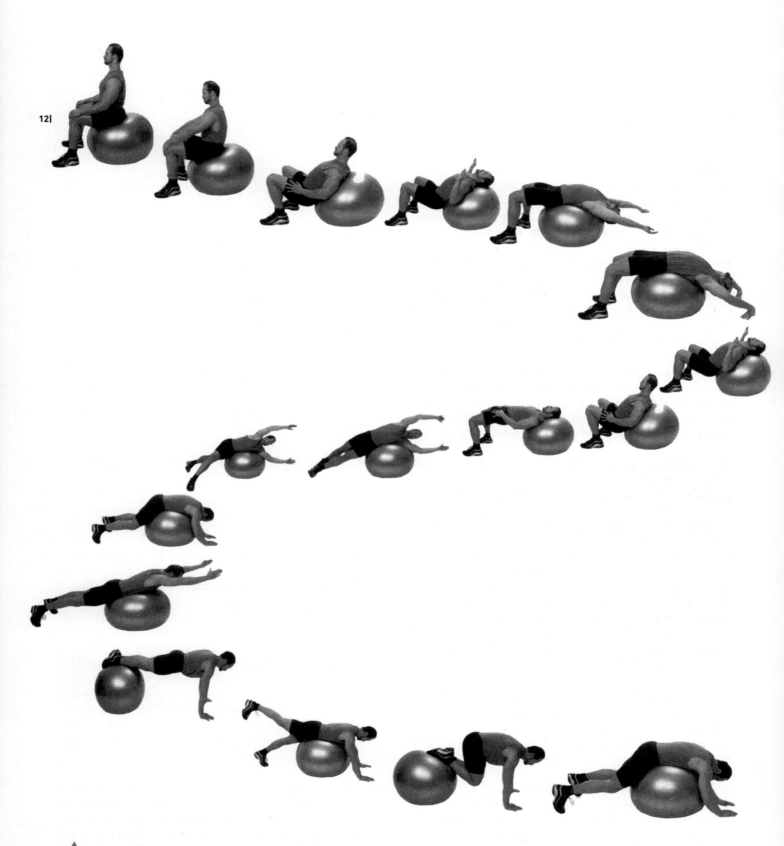

Figure 1-10 StrongPosture™ Motion on the Ball exercise flow

changes have been documented from exercise focused on improving an individual's core strength and control[xvi].

On the other hand, not only does a slump make you look and feel old before your time, but bad posture can actually shorten your life!

>**RESEARCH:** In 2004 a four-year study by Deborah Kado, MD[xvii] was published in the Journal of the American Geriatrics Society, showing that people with hyper-kyphotic posture (the bent-over "hunchback" appearance that is so common in the elderly after a lifetime of degenerating poor posture) had a 1.44-times higher mortality rate.

Or put another way:

Stand taller = Live longer

StrongPosture™ Exercise for Aging and Performing Well

This book will teach you how strengthening posture with 10 minutes of StrongPosture™ exercise a day can help you stand taller, feel better, and yes, actually live longer.

StrongPosture™ exercise creates an awareness of posture and, when performed daily, can stretch muscles, ligaments, and other structures that shorten with poor posture; strengthen muscles that weaken[xviii]; and help people stay active, thereby combating a litany of health issues from degenerative joint disease to cardiovascular and respiratory problems.

Stronger posture not only helps back and neck pain, but it also helps you feel better in general as you breathe deeper, reduce stress, and have more energy. Patients have told me they like doing their StrongPosture™ exercises. They report improvement with problems ranging from knee pain to headaches, and say they even feel, and sometimes look, taller and thinner.

Young or old, athlete or couch potato, maintaining StrongPosture™ with daily StrongPosture™ exercise is an intelligent LifeHabit for aging well. These posture-strengthening exercises are based on contemporary biomechanical concepts blended with ancient yoga practices and wisdom. My goal is to teach you to become conscious of your posture, and then strengthen your posture and balance with focused-motion StrongPosture™ exercises. Exercises can be done anywhere, and do not require any expensive equipment. A flat wall is necessary as a reference for erect posture, and then we introduce inexpensive, low-tech tools like exercise balls. Advanced StrongPosture™ exercise therapy using elastic bands and weights are effective, but beyond the scope of this book.

See www.bodyzone.com/resources for online and local vendors of posture strengthening tools.

Integrating StrongPosture™ into a routine ensures you get maximum benefit from every exercise you do. Professional and amateur athletes alike know they perform best when they perfect their form, and good form begins with StrongPosture ™.

If you have been living with weak, poor posture your whole life, you cannot just change it in an afternoon. It is common for people to try to "jump ahead" in the sequence of StrongPosture™ exercises before they have the core strength and coordination to optimally do the next exercise in a series.

Don't.

These StrongPosture™ exercises are designed to build on themselves, to be progressive. You want a strong foundation when erecting a building. Similarly, to improve posture, focus on one motion to master one motion at a time. Each StrongPosture™ exercise should be mastered before you progress to the next one so you can build movements "from the ground up" with controlled motion to first stabilize one part of the body as you then consciously move to another.

Focused attention to subtle movements can help find and strengthen weak links in your posture; doing them sloppily will accomplish far less or even aggravate a problem. For the next seven weeks, make a commitment to your life and take ten minutes a day without conversation, without distraction, and focus on your posture.

What this book is not:

There is no substitute for professional care. Consult your Doctor of Medicine if you have a systemic disease that may be affected by physical exertion (uncontrolled high

14| blood pressure, open surgical wounds, strokes, etc.) or other disease concerns. Consult a Doctor of Chiropractic if you think you have a disc syndrome, arthritis, nerve impingement disorders, or other biomechanical problems. Other professionals you may want to consult include a professional massage therapist and/or a StrongPosture™ exercise professional (yoga instructor, personal trainer, or someone certified in Alexander technique, Feldenkrais, or StrongPosture™ exercise rehab techniques). Exercise can be dramatically more or less effective, depending upon your form. We will discuss this in depth, but for now understand that proper form is the key to preventing injury, improving performance, and receiving positive health benefits from the exercise you do.

> **If you would like help refining your StrongPosture™ exercises, a list of certified Clinical StrongPosture™ exercise Professionals can be found online at www. bodyzone.com/CPEPs**

With or without posture awareness, there is more to good health and longevity than exercise. Eating right and receiving proper nutrition are essential, and there are vitamins, herbs, and other nutritional supplements that are beneficial. However, this is a book about StrongPosture™ exercise, and I leave the reader to consult other fine sources about diet and nutrition.

Part of the secret to keeping a body moving well with age is becoming conscious of how you sit, stand, and move. Do StrongPosture™ exercise every day, along with "checking in" with your posture periodically. Learning how to sit, stand, and move more intelligently (biomechanically speaking) will help you feel good today and stay active as you age.

Some words before beginning any new exercise program

Just as a rusty hinge may squeak, when you first move your body in unaccustomed patterns of motion while learning StrongPosture™ exercises you may feel a tightness or stretching you have not previously experienced. This is normal, and topical pain relief ointments usually provide quick relief. However, if sharp pain occurs or discomfort persists, consult a professional. Also, a trained StrongPosture™ exercise professional may suggest modifications or other customized exercises tailored to your individual posture type and clinical problems.

Whether you are a completely out-of-shape couch potato

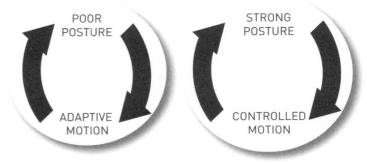

▲ **Figure 1-11** Cycle of Poor Posture vs. StrongPosture™- Strong Motion

or a trained athlete, you will likely find performing some unaccustomed motions awkward. Unused muscles are difficult to exercise. You may feel like you can't move like **THIS**, so instead you substitute a similar, but different, motion and do **THAT**. The problem is, **THAT** is usually part of the problem, and **THIS** is exactly what you need to do. The most effective way to improve posture and body motion is build a strong foundation and strengthen the core by systematically and incrementally stretching and working muscles and mobilizing joints to create new patterns of motion.

Perfect StrongPosture™ Exercises for the rest of us: PeelBacks and Progressions

Everyone is not equal, biomechanically speaking, and we don't all move the same way. Some motions and exercises are easier for some than others, but the overarching goal for anyone doing StrongPosture™ exercise should be to do the exercise perfectly *for their body*. If you cannot do an exercise perfectly (e.g., if you have to bend your knees even a little when they should be straight, or if you need to throw your arms out a bit to balance, etc.) then do a PeelBack for that exercise. PeelBacks are modifications to something you can do perfectly. With practice you can progress and ultimately strengthen a motion you initially could not do well. Then, once an exercise can be performed optimally, Progressions are more difficult variations to further challenge and strengthen balance, control, and function.

A LifeHabit is something you do consistently throughout

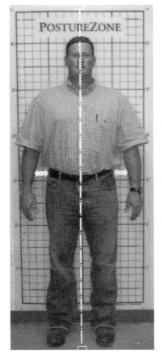

POSTUREZONE

Every journey has a beginning, and becoming conscious of your posture today is the first step to improving posture tomorrow. This exercise is deceptively difficult because it involves conscious focusing, something many of us do not often do. I jokingly call it StrongPosture™ exercise 0, because it isn't a part of a daily StrongPosture™ exercise protocol, but it should be a part of everyone's life.

◀ **Figure 1-12** Standing Normal Front View Posture

Stand up straight and be perfectly still, with your best posture, eyes looking forward, and:

> **1»** Be conscious of where your head, shoulders, and pelvis are in space.

> **2»** Be conscious of your hands and feet.

Look at a blank wall, without a mirror, for 30 seconds or so (don't look at a clock, just count 5 slow breaths). The goal is to set an image in your conscious mind of where your body is in space when you believe you are standing up straight, with your best posture.

your life. Especially if you haven't been physically active, creating a new LifeHabit of daily StrongPosture™ exercise is a great way to begin making a change. But fit or flabby, StrongPosture™ and full range motion can create a virtuous cycle to help everything move better.

Read this book from the beginning and do each exercise presented **in order.** (If you are one of those people who insist on reading the last page first, or want to see a "sample" daily StrongPosture™ exercise progression, I refer you to Appendix: Conscious StrongPosture™ exercises–Wall Protocol.) Otherwise, read a chapter and add a new exercise every few days. You will get the most benefit from learning **and practicing** these exercises on a daily basis, adding more to your sequences as your hips unflex, your shoulders roll back, your head elevates, and your posture strengthens.

Teaching patients Conscious StrongPosture™ exercises and techniques has convinced me that many of the motion problems and premature aging of our sitting society are not inevitable. Many people who first consulted me for a flare-up of their "regular" pain credit their increased postural awareness for a large part of their positive results, which is why they continue doing their exercises long after they continue to be pain-free.

»TRY THIS: *Mirror Posture Truths*

Once you have noted your best posture, see if the mirror agrees.
> Stand in front of a mirror with your eyes closed with your best posture.
> Then, open your eyes and note:
> Are you standing as straight as you thought you were?

Now relax your posture and stand normally.
> Note any additional distortions in your normal posture.

Before continuing on to the next chapter

Find Your Best Posture

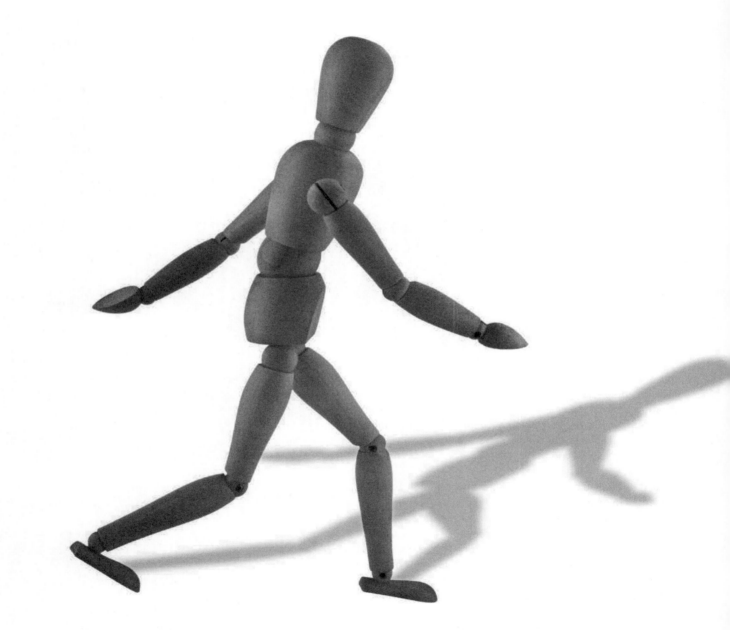

2 Posture- Where You Really Are

A chain is no stronger than its weakest link, and life is after all a chain.
William James (1842-1910)

Conscious vs. Unconscious Posture

Posture awareness is the beginning of strengthening posture. When I mention posture, people commonly tell me they know they have bad posture and then try and do what grandma advised, attempting to "stand straight," or "put your shoulders back." This usually works for about thirty seconds, until the mind wanders and they once again slouch into their familiar round-backed, forward-head slump.

Our posture is mostly unconscious. We can focus on and be conscious of posture for a few minutes at best, but the vast majority of our waking hours are spent thinking about things other than posture.

If you know you're standing straight, with good posture, does that mean you really are? Posture is quite literally how you balance your body. There are infinite combinations of possible alignments of the joints that result in a body balancing. However, there are far more combinations that result in a body falling down.

StrongPosture™ is the best biomechanical alignment of the body where all the muscles and joints are ideally aligned to work their best while stressing the body the least.

Many posture problems begin in the space between perceptions (where we think we are) and true, objective reality (where we really are). So, the first step in strengthening posture is to become aware of where we are.

Balance- Where You Really Are

Your posture is how you balance your body, so the strength of your balance is how well you know, and can control, where your body is in space. The one-leg balance test demonstrates how balance weakens as posture degenerates[xix].

One-leg balance exercises are tools to align our internal perceptions of posture with external reality. When one-leg balance is worse on one side than the other, there is unbalanced muscle function and joint stress. One study of older people showed older people who could not balance on one leg had more than twice the risk of being injured in a fall[xx].

People with poor posture and those with low-back pain usually have weak balance. On at least one (but commonly both) sides, they cannot "keep their balance." Not surprisingly, after I adjust a patient, not only do they tell me they feel better, but they often are able to balance better and even "feel lighter." Since a stressed posture requires more energy to keep upright and move through space this makes sense.

The first step in creating posture awareness is observing how long, and how well, you can balance on one leg.

»TRY THIS: *One - Leg Balance Test*

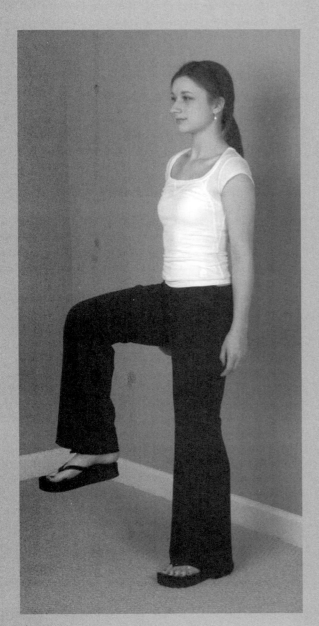

The **STANDING ONE-LEG BALANCE** test compares your perception of where you think you are in space with the true reality of where you are.

1. Stand up straight and lift your left knee so your foot comes off the ground. Slowly count and stop the first time you have to put your foot down or wave your arms to balance. (Don't cheat!)

2. Repeat on the other side.

3. How long can you balance on your left leg? On your right one?

You should be able to balance on each leg for at least twenty seconds. If you cannot, either you are not where you think you are when you are standing straight, or your muscles are too weak to keep you in one place for that long. In any event, your body is not functioning as well as it could. Especially if you find yourself twisting, throwing your arms out, or otherwise dancing about to balance on one foot, you're demonstrating signs of weak balance. Do not be discouraged! In fact, congratulations are in order, since being conscious of a problem is the first step to change.

▲ **Figure 2-1** One - leg balance

201

StrongPosture™ Balance:

The Stork- 30 Seconds to Strong Balance

"The single best exercise that can be done anytime, without any special equipment, is nothing more complicated than standing on one foot for as long as possible and then switching to the other foot."
Richard Restak, noted author and researcher

If you don't balance, you fall down!
The Stork is a variation of a basic yoga posture, and is as simple as just standing up straight and lifting your foot. Then all you have to do is not fall down.

However, as with many things in StrongPosture™ exercise (and life, for that matter) when you look at the details, things are not as easy as they appear.

If you cannot stand on one leg as well as the other there is a weakness or imbalance somewhere in your kinetic chain of posture, StrongPosture™ exercises such as the Stork strengthen and train the less-used anti-gravity muscles to strengthen balance.

■ **First, show me your best posture**

- Stand up with your best posture, looking straight in front of you.
  - Be conscious of where your head, shoulders, and pelvis are in space.
- Keep your best posture.
- Lift your right knee so it is at 90°.
  - Thigh should be parallel to the floor and level so you can balance a pencil and
    - Foot is under your knee, and
    - Toes point forward.

■ **Stand straight and focus on your best StrongPosture™ for 30 seconds**

- Keep your left knee locked and perfectly straight

- **Don't hyper-extend (i.e., don't move the knee backward)**
- **Even a slight knee bend is cheating.**

To keep your balance don't:

> Wave your arms
> Twist
> Dance/hop around

■ **Repeat, with the left leg.**

In order to be effective, StrongPosture™ exercises should be done perfectly for your body. If you can't stand straight for 30 seconds, put your foot down, take a breath or two, focus, and try again twice more. It is far better to work the correct but unused muscles for a few seconds than to work the incorrect muscles for hours.

Do the Stork three times a day (or more if you like).

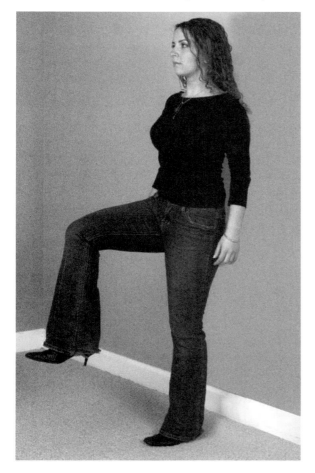

▲ **Figure 2-2** Strong One - leg posture

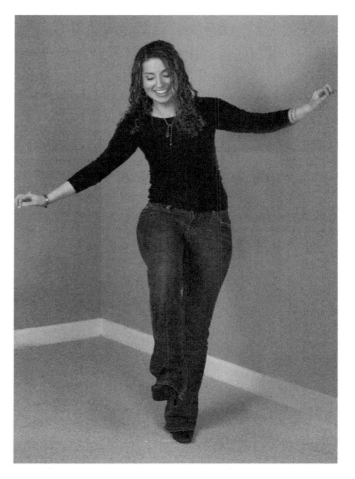

▲ **Figure 2-3** Weak One-leg balance

PEELBACKS

22|

If you can't stand with your best posture for 30 seconds without falling over, swinging your arms, or "dancing" to keep your balance, try these StrongPosture™ exercise PeelBacks.

PEELBACK: The Flamingo (Especially good for geriatrics and people with injuries)

Stand with StrongPosture ™.
Press your left foot into the ground--lock the knee.
If you can't lock it fully straight, make it as straight as it goes pain free.

> Then, keep StrongPosture™ as you lift your right foot.
> Bend the right knee slightly so the right toe is next to the left ankle.
> Keep your shoulders and hips square and level.

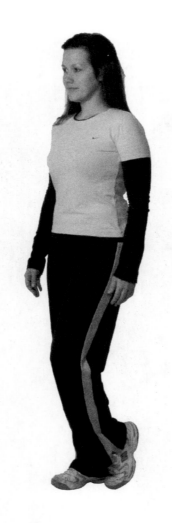

▲ **Figure 2-4** The Flamingo

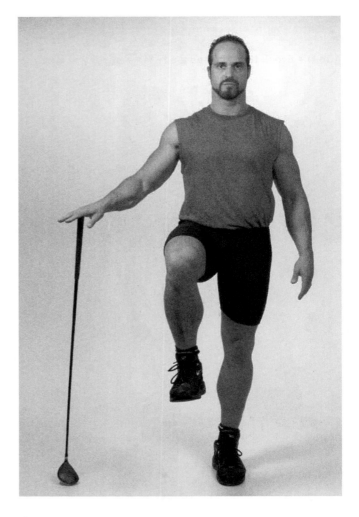

▲ **Figure 2-5** Supported Stork One - leg balance

PEELBACK: *Supported Stork One-leg Balance*

Use a walking stick, wall or the back of a chair to stabilize.

• First stand up with StrongPosture ™.
• Then touch a wall to stabilize. Lift your right leg and keep StrongPosture ™. Repeat on the left side.

After a few days, try and take your hand away for a few seconds while maintaining StrongPosture ™. Gradually lengthen the time you are standing without touching the wall.

You are far better off standing on one foot for 5 seconds with StrongPosture™ while touching the wall than dancing on one foot for 30 seconds. In order to be effective, StrongPosture™ exercises should be done perfectly for your body. Your individual posture type and history of injury will affect how your body balances, but if you can help it balance better, it can age better.

PEELBACK: *Leg Up*

If you cannot raise your knee and balance, instead of lifting your knee, keep your thigh down and just bend your knee and lift your foot just so your leg is behind you.

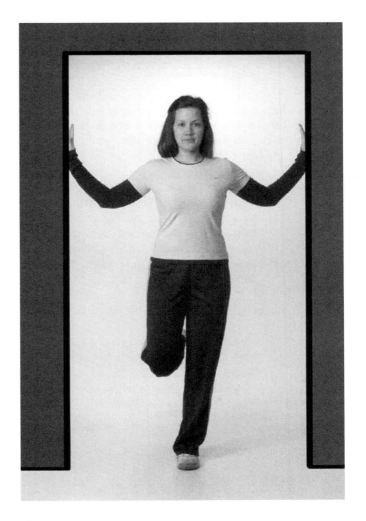

▲ **Figure 2-6** Leg - up balance with support

Work up to balancing for 30 seconds on each leg, 3 times a day, with StrongPosture™. Build Strong Balance by standing on one leg as you wait for coffee to brew, wait in line, or even when you are brushing your teeth.

PROGRESSIONS:

• Over time, try to increase up to 60 seconds while maintaining your best posture.
Remember: only progress as long as you can keep your perfect form. Only do what you can do well.
• Start to be aware of your breathing as you balance on one leg.
• Slowly put your arms over your head, then back down back at your side. Repeat, but this time lift your arms to the sides and back down.
• Close your eyes for 5 seconds. Then try it for 10 seconds.

•Closing your eyes takes away visual input, leaving your brain only information from the ears (vestibular) and joint receptors to balance. Just as a weightlifter increases the weight to strengthen muscles, unused nerve pathways strengthen when you depend upon their input to effectively balance.

The Clock: visualize yourself in the middle of a clock.

Then, while balancing on one foot:
Hop toward 12, then return to the center.
Repeat, but hop to 6 o'clock.
Then stop at every quarter hour.
Stop at every hour.

Breath Focus Progression:

Do the Stork and while focusing on your breathing for 5 slow, deep breaths

Push your stomach out as you breathe in
Pull your stomach in as you breathe out

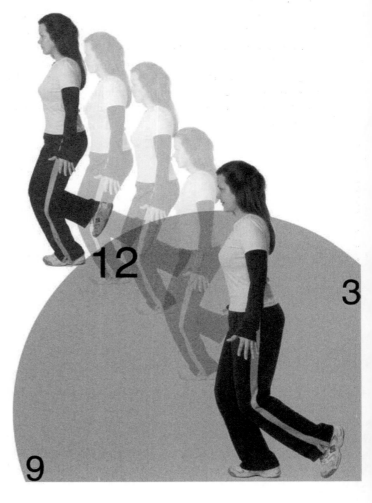

▲ **Figure 2-7** One - leg Clock Hop

Looking at Your Posture: Aligning Perceptions and Reality

If you are observant, you can see a lot. Yogi Berra

Earlier you made a mental note of your "best" posture (if you haven't done this yet, stand up, find a mirror, and do so now).

When I talk about posture, the first question many people have is "How's my posture?" I'm always amazed at how unaware people are of their posture! Many people tell me they know they have poor posture, but then claim that they can stand straight "when they want to." However, when we take their posture picture, despite their best efforts to stand up straight, they are surprised to see how distorted their posture appears. Perception and reality don't always agree.

Imagine This:

Have you ever been in a plane as it is beginning to taxi away from the gate, and then realize that the plane next to yours is moving, not yours? Or thinking your car is moving forward and being startled when you realize the car next to you is backing up? Regardless of your perceptions, reality is.

Our sitting lifestyle forces us to balance our bodies in ways that stress muscles and joints, and have created an epidemic of muscle and joint problems. Some people non-judgmentally accept poor posture thinking, "That is just the way I am." Perhaps it's partly because we, the people of the early 21st century, are all children of the late 20th century when the prevailing philosophy was relativism, leading to "Do your own thing," because "Everything is relative." Classroom emphasis on posture disappeared, and the stereotypical mother and grandmother who admonished kids to "stand straight" became far more rare. Perhaps part of the blame for poor posture should be on society. Our psychological pendulum swung away from making judgments based on unthinking prejudice and toward compassion for our fellows, creating ideas such as "I'm OK, you're OK." And for many facets of society, this has been a wonderful thing. People should be judged as individuals, not on preconceptions or bigotries. Tremendous good has occurred as a result of society's newfound tolerance and understanding.

However, being judgmental is not always a bad thing. Along with many other things, posture isn't relative. Since it must obey the laws of physics, mechanically speaking there is good posture and there is poor posture.

Some people contend that pain is all in the mind, and, to some degree, this is true. However, while the pain from a brick being dropped on your foot may be in your head, the tissue damage is real. If the brick fractures your toe, the resulting limp from the pain will have an equally real effect on the rest of your body (as well as putting your mind in a really bad mood).

One way to view the mechanics of posture is to compare balancing the segments of your body to a child's stack of blocks. When the blocks are all balanced, the stack is stable. But when one is out of place, the blocks above are wobbly. To most effectively balance a stack of blocks, you put the second block as squarely as you can on top of the first. Then, you

26| squarely place the third block on the second, because it can only be as stable as the blocks below. And so on.

A posture distortion or misalignment may be the cause, the effect, or a cause of another effect further up, or down, the chain of body motion. Since the body must balance, a posture distortion may be the area of initial injury, or a result of the body compensating to maintain balance. An injury to the knees, ankles, or feet can force the body to maintain balance by compensating with hyper-extended knees (i.e., moving the knees backward), which in turn causes knee weakness and wear. Simple principles—that the body must balance, that it compensates, moves in patterns, and adapts—can cause myriad biomechanical problems. So if we want to strengthen posture, the first step is to align our postural perceptions with true reality.

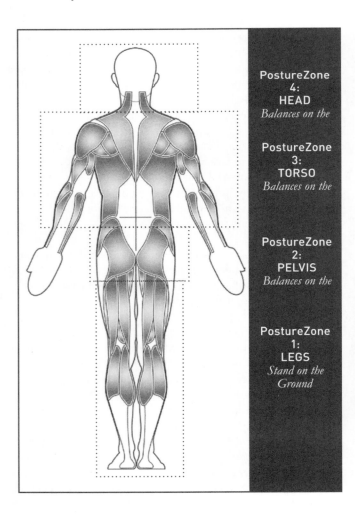

PostureZone
4:
HEAD
Balances on the

PostureZone
3:
TORSO
Balances on the

PostureZone
2:
PELVIS
Balances on the

PostureZone
1:
LEGS
*Stand on the
Ground*

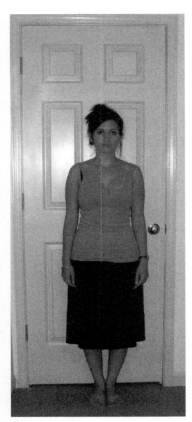

Figure 2-8b Six panel doors work well as a reference grid for posture pictures

Figure 2-8a Building blocks of posture

Checking in with Reality:
Taking a Posture Picture

Man will become better only when you make him see what he is like. Anton Chekhov

Mention posture and people shift about and pull their shoulders back to "stand straight." When they do, some people may feel tightness in the shoulders, while others may feel tightness in their legs, their low back, or wherever the tight link is in *their* body's chain of motion.

The best place to begin finding the tight link is by using our eyes. Looking at posture gives a tremendous amount of information about how a body is working. However, the overlapping causes and effects of a lifetime's habits and injuries make assessment an art as well as a science.

In the "Find Your Best Posture" demo you took a mental "picture" of your best posture. Now we are going to use a camera to create a baseline—your postural starting point.

Get a digital camera (or a Polaroid if you are old-fashioned) and a friend to help. Have your friend take two photographs of your posture, one from the front and one from the side. It doesn't matter which side, but we usually have people face to their right for uniformity and so we can easily compare before and after pictures.

The person being photographed should stand against a background with at least one objective vertical reference, such as a window frame or a door. Clinically we use a PostureGrid, but six-panel doors can work as a grid at home for an objective background. Also, close fitting clothes show better details of alignment.

> **Note:** The assessments of back (or posterior) posture images are beyond the scope of this book, but if you are feeling ambitious by all means also take a picture of your best posture from the back. Theoretically you should look symmetrical, with your spine centered. If not, almost all of the asymmetries you see from the back will have effects visible from the front and side as well. A Clinical StrongPosture™ exercise Professional (CPEP) can help you assess a back view of your body.
> **See www.BodyZone.com/CPEPs.**

Instructions to photographer:

In a well-lighted area, stand about 6-8 feet away from your subject. Hold the camera level with the ground (a tripod is helpful but not at all necessary).
Frame the picture so you can see the person's entire body, from the toes to the top of the head.

Now, read the following to the person whose posture you are photographing.

Instructions to person whose posture is being checked:

> Stand normally.
> Look straight ahead.
> Relax, and don't stand unnaturally.
> Now, Find Your Best Posture.

Take one picture from the front, and then repeat from the side.

IF YOU DON'T HAVE A CAMERA AVAILABLE:

> Look at your posture from the front view by using a full-length mirror.

Standing in front of the mirror, first

> - Close your eyes,
> Then
> - Stand straight with your best posture, then, without moving,
> - Open your eyes and observe your posture.

▌Assessing Your Posture Picture

Look closely at each picture. The building blocks of posture are the head, the shoulders, the arms, the torso, the pelvis, and lower extremity. When considering the questions below, if the answer is not yes, ask yourself: What is out of alignment?

Front View Posture Picture Assessment

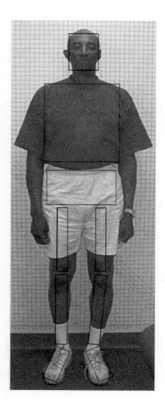

▲ **Figure 2-9** Front view ideals

•We balance from the bottom up, so look at your posture picture from the bottom up and note:

> •Is the pelvis level and symmetrically centered over the knees and ankles?
> •Are the shoulders and chest level on top of the pelvis?
> •Is the head level on top of the chest?

•Can you draw a vertical line down the middle of your body so it's evenly spaced between the eyes, middle chest, belly button, and then evenly between both legs?

• **NOTES**

> •Right-handed people usually have a low right shoulder and high right hip.
> •Left-handed people usually have a low left shoulder and high left hip.
> •Scoliosis (spinal curvature) is a common congenital problem that can cause a high shoulder on one side and a high hip on the other.
> •Side-to-side distortions are common results of adaptations from major and minor injuries and habits such as
>> • carrying a purse on one side,
>> • talking on a phone using one shoulder for a cradle,
>> • or habitually sitting on a fat wallet in a hip pocket, etc.

• **Is one foot turned out?**

> • If so, march in place for 7 steps and re-check.
>> •If the foot is still turned out, there may be a sacroiliac or other distortion of the pelvis.

PostureZone 1: Lower extremity

• **Are the knees, ankles, and feet angled the same on both sides?**

•Does one foot, ankle or knee face differently than its partner? Asymmetrical motion not only stresses and strains the feet, ankles, knees, but stress goes up the spine.

• **Are the soles of the shoes worn evenly?**

Poor foot posture alters the leg biomechanics and so shoes wear unevenly as well as different from one side to the other

A common problem affecting many people is feet that roll in, or pronate. A pronated foot has a prominent ankle on the inside, and a sunken one on the outside from the body's weight rolling over the inside edge of the foot.

Pronators usually benefit from a customized insert for their shoes called an orthotic. Prescription orthotics are manufactured from a cast of your foot, usually taken by a chiropractor, podiatrist or physical therapist. However, many people get a lot of relief from over the counter generic shoe inserts now available online and at specialty shoe care retailers.

Pronators usually wear out their shoes unevenly, with the outside edge of the heel being worn, while the inside edge is like new. This counter-intuitive wear pattern results from the way the pronating foot strikes the ground while walking or running. Also, uneven pronation adds further stress as the muscles on the over-pronated side overwork and shorten over time in response to working harder against gravity. When you see an over-pronated foot, the muscles on that side are usually tight.

• **Shoe wear and orthotics**
Almost all serious athletes, and especially runners, note that their shoes wear more evenly when they use orthotics to balance the biomechanical function of their feet.

PostureZone 2: Pelvis

• **Is the pelvis shifted to one side?**

•Indicates tightness or imbalance of the thigh muscles (aka TFL) or weakness of the deep hip muscles (aka gluteus medius).

PostureZone 3: Torso

• **Are the arms and hands spaced evenly from the body on both sides?**

•If one arm is touching the body and one is not, or if the arms are not equally spaced from the body, then either the shoulders are not over the pelvis (as discussed above), or the shoulders are not sitting on the chest symmetrically. Uneven carriage of the shoulders can result from always sleeping on the same side or work habits. The school bus driver who always uses one arm to push the handle to open a door, the carpenter who always hammers with his right hand, and the secretary who always reaches the same awkward way to use her mouse in a poorly designed workstation are all training their body to have weak posture.

• **Can you see the backs of either (or both) hands?**

•When standing straight, you should only see the thumb side of the hands, with back of the hands and the pinky finger hidden behind the hand. If you can see the backs of the hands, it usually means the shoulders are rounded forward. This is a very common observation, especially when there is a Forward Head Posture observed from the side view.

30|

Side View Posture Picture Assessment

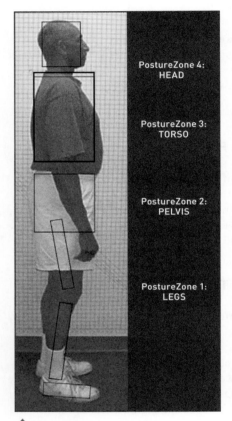

PostureZone 4:
HEAD

PostureZone 3:
TORSO

PostureZone 2:
PELVIS

PostureZone 1:
LEGS

▲ **Figure 2-10** Side view ideals

Remember: The body is always balancing. When looking at a body from the side, the question to ask yourself is, "How?" Noting what is moved forward and what is moved back in order to balance can give tremendous insight into someone's habits and past injuries, as well as their current problems and complaints. Observe the following and consider:

How is the body shifting its weight in order to balance?
How does the resulting compensation and adaptation affect the front contour of the body?
How does the resulting compensation and adaptation affect the back contour of the body?

Look at the side-view picture, from the bottom up, and note:

PostureZone 1:

■ Lower extremity: Are the hips, knees, and feet aligned?

•**NOTE:** are the hips above knees, and the knees above, or just slightly forward, of the ankles?
•In neutral posture, the thighs and calves should be roughly vertical.

PostureZone 2:

■ Pelvis: Are the hips level, or is the pelvis tilted forward, or backward? Does the belly protrude?

•There is dramatic postural difference between how a person stands when the pelvis is level, and when they are arching back because the pelvis is tilting forward. Especially when someone is overweight, the pelvis tilts forward.
•Not all people with protruding abdomens are overweight. Many people in good shape have a protruding abdomen, and roll their pelvis forward. Fit or fat, the body has to balance.
•Forward tilts also occur from folding the body in a sitting posture as the muscles in front of the hips (the flexors) shorten and the muscles behind the hips (the extensors) lengthen.
•If someone has tight hip flexors, a rolled-in chest, or other common posture distortion, they must compensate and adapt. A protruding abdomen pulls the pelvis forward, rolling the pelvis into a forward tilt. When the pelvis rolls forward, the shoulders and torso go back to keep you from falling onto your face. The head then juts forward to compensate and balance.
• A flat stomach is the holy grail of fitness. Late night TV ads promise that you too can have "six-pack, washboard abs" if you buy an ab-rollers, belly blaster, six-pack cutter, or other exercise contraption, lotion, or potion. So why do many people who are in good shape still work unsuccessfully to have a flat stomach? The answer is frequently in their posture.

PostureZone 3:

■ Torso: Are the shoulders level and even with the hips?

•Your posture is how you balance your body, so if your shoulders are not over your hips, you are working harder than you should to hold yourself up. Many people who complain of "tired backs" have reported dramatic relief after learning to balance with stronger posture. Of course, this means you have to become conscious of your posture, which is one very good reason to take a side-view picture.

■ Arms: Are the arms resting at the side, with the back of the hand visible?
  • Is the chest elevated or depressed?
  • Is the pinky side of the hand hiding the thumb?
  Forward, rolled in shoulders frequently accompany Forward Head Posture because in our society people keep their hands close together to type, drive, write and do many other modern tasks. When the arms are in front of the body the shoulders are rolled forward and the chest depresses, making it hard to take a deep breath as the shoulders follow our hands and eyes forward into the classic rounded shoulder, forward head posture.

PostureZone 4:
■ Head: Is the head level and balanced above the shoulders?

  •Forward head posture (FHP) is an epidemic in our society, and is arguably the most common and problematic posture adaptation. Forward head posture causes chronic problems such neck pain, headaches, and arm pain and contributes to conditions ranging from osteoarthritis in the neck to carpal tunnel syndrome.
  •For every inch that the head moves forward of the torso, the weight of the head carried by the lower neck and upper back doubles. The computer worker, the student, and Joe Average sitting round-backed in his recliner, have all trained their bodies to balance despite this increased biomechanical stress and strain. The predictable result is adaptive overwork and tightness of some neck, upper back, and shoulder muscles; atrophy of other muscles, and over time, premature spinal degeneration.

32|

Body Contour Observations- Look at the front of the body

■ PostureZone 1: Lower Extremity: Are the feet the most forward part of the body?
■ PostureZone 2: Pelvis: Is the pelvis level (normal) or tilted forward?

  • Head: Is the head forward of the chest?
  • Is the nose and are the ears level (normal) or is the nose pointing upward?

Is the belly large and protruding, pulling the pelvis forward?
■ PostureZone 3: Torso:
  • Shoulders: Are they square (normal) or do they roll in?
  Is the chest depressed?
  • Arms: Are the palms flat against the side of the thigh (normal), or are they in front of the body?

■ PostureZone 4: Head: Is the head forward of the chest?
  • Is the nose and are the ears level (normal) or is the nose pointing upward?

Body Contour Observations- Look at the back of the body

■ PostureZone 1: Lower Extremity: Are the knees straight or locked back (hyper-extended)?
■ PostureZone 2: Pelvis: Does the low back arch more than normal? Does the low back curve forward (swayback) or flatten (flat back)? Are the buttocks rounded or flat, or tilted forward or back?
■ Posture Zone 3: Torso:
  • Shoulders: Is there an increased "humping" of the middle back?
  Indicates adaptive shortening of important posture muscles, including the latissimus dorsi(lats), pectorals, and psoas.
  • Are the shoulders rounded?
  •Do the shoulder blades wing out?
    Usually caused by weakness of deep shoulder muscles (serratus anterior, pectorals and mid to lower trapezius).
  • Arms: Are the palms flat against the side of the thigh, or are they on the front of the thigh? Can you see the pinky?
    If not, then the arms are rotated internally (rolled in).
■ Posture Zone 4: Head: Is the head forward of the chest?

If you don't like what you see when you look at your posture, or you see that you are not standing as straight you thought you were, you are not alone. If you haven't taken a picture of your posture yet, I encourage you strongly to do this simple exercise.

Becoming conscious of your posture is the beginning of making a positive change. When you do, consider making a copy of each image—Place one in this book, and one someplace you see everyday such as on your bathroom mirror or refrigerator. Once you know where you are, then you can begin improving.

REMEMBER:

Being conscious of a problem is the first step to change.

Finding Your Balance on the Ball

Exercise balls, available at any sporting goods store, can be uniquely valuable tools to help you become conscious of, and improve, posture and body motion. Simply sitting on a ball trains deep core muscles in your spine and throughout your body to move and support you in new ways.

When sitting or exercising on a ball, you must balance. If you don't balance, you fall off the ball. When you start to fall, we can say you have bad balance, or we can see that our inner subjective perceptions and true reality disagree. The feeling of "falling off the ball" provides feedback to the brain, as well as the position sense receptors in the muscles and joints, which begins the process of aligning an individual's perceived and true postural reality.

> *Ball exercises align our perceptions with true reality.*
> *First, by helping us find unbalanced motion, and*
> *Then, specifically exercising ways to improve it.*

Exercising on an unstable ball forces you to use your core muscles to balance, or you fall off. Requiring a body to balance differently as it is exercising sends a concentration of signals to the brain, retraining learned motion patterns. Conscious effort is required at first, but with training new unconscious motion programs develop which prevent injury by speeding reflex reactions to unanticipated stresses on the body[xxi]. Also, StrongPosture™ exercise not only improves balance, but helps strengthen lower extremity muscles, showing faster gains than weights, machines, or other forms of isotonic strength training[xxii].

Choosing the Right Ball

Ball Height

Since we usually sit with our knees at a 90° knee angle it is usually best to do so when exercising on a ball and target unused core muscle fibers. Sit about a third of the way back on a ball with your thighs level.

Many exercise balls on the market suggest a ball based upon your height. This usually ends up with a ball that is far too low for most people to comfortably sit on for any period of time.

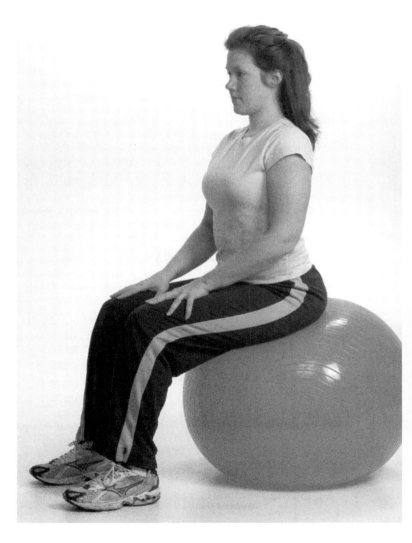

▲ **Figure 2-11** Balancing on a ball with thighs level

34|

Inflation

A good ball should be firm, not rigid (follow manufacturer's instructions on inflation).

General Exercise Advice

Balls are safe EXCEPT IF YOU FALL OFF.

Don't exercise near sharp objects (e.g., corners of glass tables, fireplace tools, etc.).

Consider investing in a yoga mat, but in any event carpet is better than hardwood, and tile or concrete can be a bad idea.

If you are unsure about your stability, try sitting on a ball facing into a corner, using the walls to brace yourself.

In other words, **USE COMMON SENSE**. If you have a bad reaction to a ball exercise including but not limited to difficulty breathing, chest pain, dizziness, vertigo (the room is spinning), severe headache, numbness, burning, loss of sensation in any part of the body, nausea, fever, or feeling uncomfortably hot, then **STOP!**

ALSO, if it hurts, back off. Over time you will learn to tell the difference between the good pain of working the body in new ways, and the bad pain of tissue injury.

IF YOU AREN'T SURE...STOP and consult a physician or trainer!!

StrongPosture™ Balance: ## BallSit

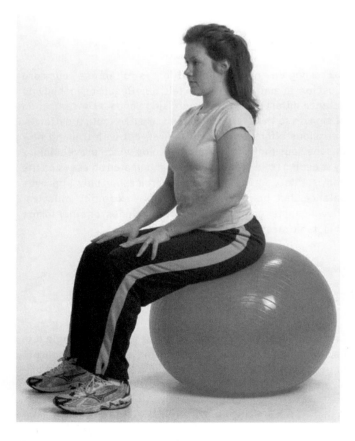

▲ **Figure 2-12** BallSit with StrongPosture ™

Goals:

- Becoming conscious of balance.

- Feeling the difference between where you think your body is and where your body truly is in space.
- Getting comfortable on the ball.

BallSit Aware Posture

It may be helpful to have a partner read the following part to you out loud as you sit on the ball:

Begin by simply sitting on the ball. In order to balance, you must unconsciously activate the deep core muscles of the torso. Roll the ball around a bit and get comfortable and notice: Are you slumped over or sitting erect?

Now, be aware: Sit up straight.

StrongPosture™ begins from the bottom up.
Starting with the lower body, pull and tighten the feet, knees, and pelvis in a StrongPosture™ position.

> Place your feet hip distance apart and square on the floor.
> Many people roll their ankles in (pronation), so you may have to roll the ankles slightly out so all four corners of the feet are squarely and equally weighted and grounded.
> Check to be sure both knees are at 90°, with the heel directly beneath the knee, and the calf vertical.
> Next, roll the shoulders back and down, pulling the tips of the shoulder blades together with the hands on thighs, palms up.
> Next, as you look straight ahead, pull the head directly over the shoulders by gently pulling the neck back (keep your head level)
> Some people may feel like they are tucking their head down
> Now take 5 slow belly breaths.

To strengthen posture, we must align the body as we exercise. Training strong, conscious posture and core strength is not just a ten-minute-a-day StrongPosture™ exercise, but should be integrated with other exercises so we have the strength, flexibility, endurance, and coordination to resist the forces that can cause potential injuries and to optimize sports performance.

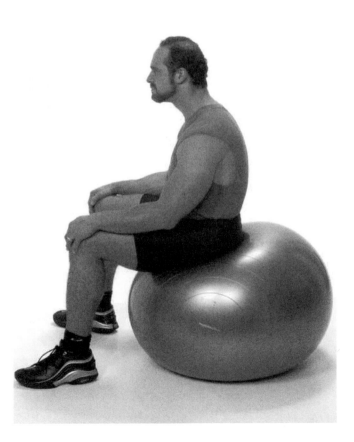

▲ **Figure 2-13** BallSit with weak posture

³⁶| **BallSit Conscious Motion**

With StrongPosture™, shoulders and arms square –
Move the ball around, first front and back, and then to the
left, then the right.
Now try to keep the ball as still as you can and move your
arms and shoulders.
Then bend forward and touch the floor.
Then do a side bend and touch the floor to your left, and
then right.
Repeat each movement three times.

PEELBACKS:

For more stability:
     Spread your feet farther apart.
     Hold your thighs with your hands
          or if you must, hold the ball

PROGRESSIONS:

Once you perfect a motion, try these ideas to refine your
form and challenge deep muscles.
However, you want listen to your body. Only add new exercises
as you gain control and improved fluidity, and never progress
past your point of comfort.

BallSit Focus

Put your feet together when you are sitting on the ball, heels
and toes touching.
Then, keeping your feet together, do a BallSit while holding
your arms out to the side.
     Then, rotate your arms in small circles, first forward,
     then backward, 10 times.

To strengthen muscles in all directions, imagine you are in
the center of a clock, and roll the ball so you touch all the
numbers.

Use your hips to write your name with the ball.

Then write numbers from 1-10.

Then write the alphabet.

Try a BallSit twist.

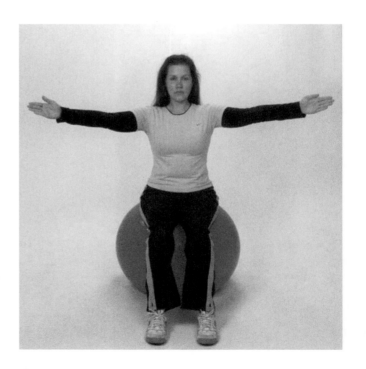

▲ **Figure 2-14** BallSit forward arm roll

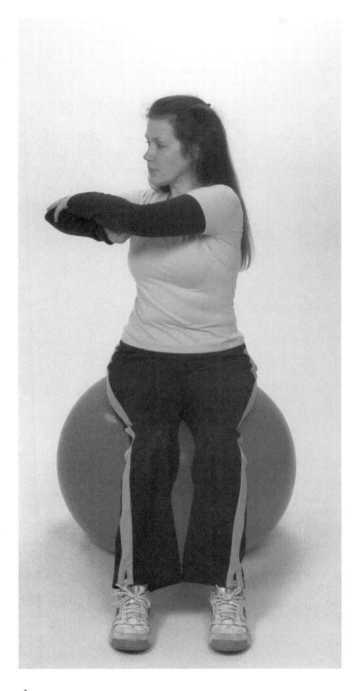

▲ **Figure 2-15** BallSit twist

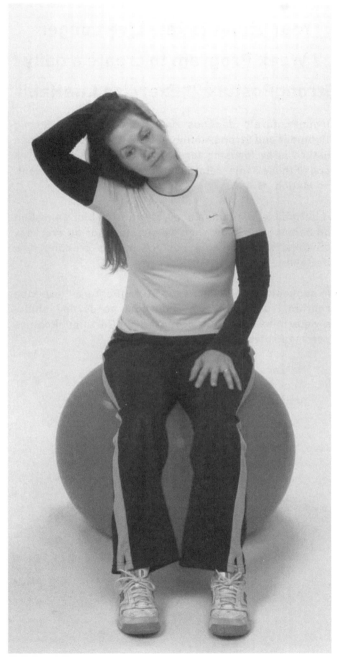

▲ **Figure 2-16** BallSit neck stretch

Try some neck stretches and rolls.

38|

B.A.M

Your Stand Taller~Live Longer
7 Week Program to create a daily
StrongPosture™ Exercise LifeHabit

StrongPosture™ depends on Strong Balance, Strong Alignment and Strong Motion. The best way to strengthen posture is by focusing for a few moments each day on each of these 3 interrelated factors- Balance, Alignment, and Motion- B.A.M.

A LifeHabit is just that, a habit of your life. Since we align and balance our body when we sit, stand, or do everyday activities, strengthening posture means creating new LifeHabits.

We suggest the following daily StrongPosture™ exercise program (subject to your individual needs and ability as determined by your physician or Certified Posture Exercise Professional (CPEP)):

> Balance focus 3 times a day.
> Alignment focus 2 times a day.
> Motion focus once a day.

Strong Balance: Do One-leg balance (the Stork) at least 3 times a day.
Strong Alignment: Do BallSit aware posture 2 times a day.
Strong Motion: Do BallSit conscious motion once a day.

Some exercises like the Stork you can do anytime, but for ball exercises we suggest setting a time each day to focus on StrongPosture™ and motion. Adding StrongPosture™ exercise to your daily routine is the key to making a lasting change in posture.

Make doing the Stork a habit by incorporating it into your daily activities:

- As you brush your teeth in the morning,
- While you are waiting for the coffee (or tea) to brew,
- Before sitting down to watch TV at night.

Alternatively:

- Do a modified Stork by standing on one leg with your best posture while putting on your socks (bending over as necessary).
- Try and put on your shoes while standing on one leg. Now, can you tie them?

Standing on one leg may look silly, but it helps invigorate you when you spend a lot of your time on your feet as well as waking up and strengthening the core muscles of posture. Our goal is to retrain your body and pattern new posture and motion.

An idea for BallSit Strong Motion:
If you have an office chair on rollers, try some of the BallSit exercises in your chair, rolling it about. If someone looks at you funny and asks what you are doing, just tell them you are doing your StrongPosture™ exercises!

StrongPosture™
7 Week Program-

B
A
M

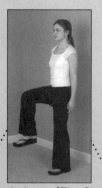

One-leg balance (**The Stork**) -p.19

Strong Balance

BALANCE

3 times a day

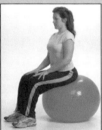

BallSit with StrongPosture™ -p.34

Strong Alignment

ALIGNMENT

2 times a day

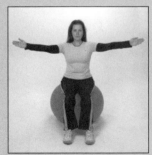

BallSit conscious motion -p.36

Strong Motion

MOTION

1 once a day

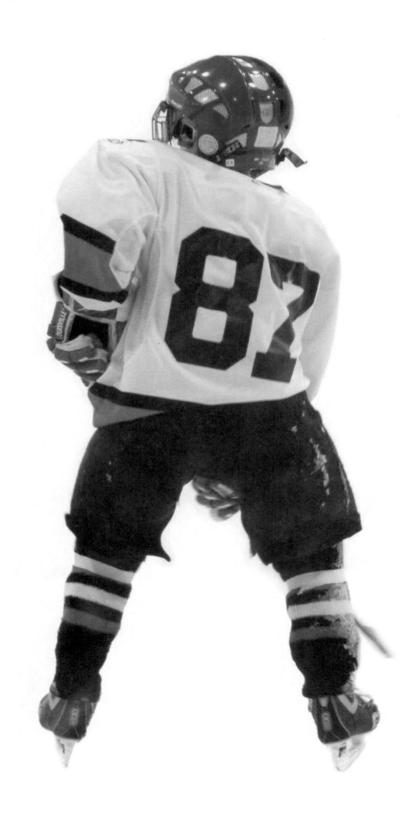

3 Posture Anatomy:

The parts of our body that we use to stand up, sit down and move around

Before we go on, let's take a look at what makes up our posture. Posture is not just how you hold your neck or the slump of your shoulders and low back. Everything in the body is connected, and our posture is the coordinated workings of all the different mechanical parts of the body.

The body's motion system controls posture. Scientists call this system the neuro-musculo-skeletal system (NMS), and break it down into three component systems[xxiii]:

42| ■ **Contracting System**

    Muscles contracting to create motion

       ■ Also called the Active System, because it requires active control

■ **Connecting System**

    The framework of the body

       ■ Also called the Passive System, because we have no active control of these tissues, which include:

    • Bones: to hold the body up.

    • Ligaments: to hold the bones together at the joints.

       ■ Joint Capsule: the ligamentous sack around every joint containing the synovial fluid for joint lubrication.

    • Tendons to hold the muscles to the bone.

    • Cartilage and discs: to protect weight-bearing and stressed surfaces where bones meet in joints.

    • Fascia: Tissue holding all the pieces together.

■ **Control System**

    Telling the muscles what to do, and when to do it

    • Brain: gives the orders, both consciously and unconsciously.

    • Spinal cord: main cable and low-level processing for information between the brain and everything in the body.

    • Nerves: the wires controlling the muscles.

    • Mechanoreceptors: sensors within muscles and joints telling the brain where the body is in space. For example, you can tell if your hand is open or clenched in a fist even without looking because of these deep sensors.

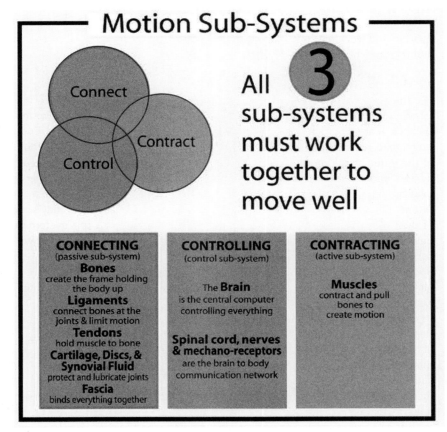

▲ **Figure 3-1** Contracting, Connecting, and Control components of the motion system

Different tissues controlling motion have different jobs and functions, but they work together and integrate to allow the complex motion we take for granted. Functionally the musculo-skeletal system and the nervous system can be looked at as one big system. So technically speaking, the Contracting, Connecting and Control systems are not true organ systems, but are actually subsystems of the neuro-musculoskeletal system.

Our bodies move when, either consciously or unconsciously, brain and nerves of the control system tell the muscles what to do, within the constraints of the physical limitations of the muscles, ligaments, and tendons. The human body is literally designed to move, and that motion follows in a chain, known as a kinetic chain. Posture and body motion depend on the coordinated workings of these Contracting, the Connecting, and the Control systems.

An individual's genetics and their current physical condition set the limit for that person's "normal posture." So, an intelligent goal is to move as best we can with what we have. Our physical structure consists of the muscles and bones, restrained by the ligaments, with muscles forming much of the outer shape of our body. Since most of us don't see perfect bodies when we look in the mirror, it is illogical to expect our posture to be perfect. No matter how hard I try to "stand up straight," I will never have the nearly ideal posture of Justin Timberlake or Angelina Jolie. The correlation between beauty and posture is supported by the fact that celebrities as varied as Sting, Julie Andrews, Paul Newman, Robin Williams, William Hurt, James Earl Jones, and Paul McCartney have been trained in posture strengthening techniques .

Posture problems are biomechanical, so finding the source of a problem requires looking at the whole body, not just at the area of pain. Injury and pain forces the muscles on the sound side of the body to overwork and compensate. Since the Contracting, Connecting, and the Control systems are links in this chain of motion, let's review the workings of each to see how they all contribute to StrongPosture™ and healthy body motion.

The Contracting System:
Muscles, the Engine of Motion

When people think of body motion, they think of muscles -for good reason: muscles move the body.

Muscles shorten (contract) to move bones & create motion.
> No matter how we are moving, no matter whether we are pushing or pulling, muscles only shorten. Muscles are like ropes: they can only pull. Every muscle has a partner muscle, known as its opposer or antagonist. In order for a muscle to lengthen, another must shorten.

The bones work as levers, and the joints act as fulcrums for the body's motion.
> Every muscle's partner pulls a bone in the opposite direction, lengthening the muscle and returning the joint to its starting position. If it weren't for its partner, we could not move our joints, because once a muscle flexed a joint, it would be stuck in that flexed position. Each muscle in a pair of muscles pulls a joint in the opposite direction. To reverse the direction of joint motion, the muscles switch roles.

Every joint is moved by many muscles. The muscles that move a part of the body often are not directly over that part. Some muscles only move a single joint, others move multiple joints. The overall motion of the body is a result of the combination of these interdependent, combined motions.
> The muscles that move the fingers are in the upper forearm, but are connected to the fingers by tendons.

44|

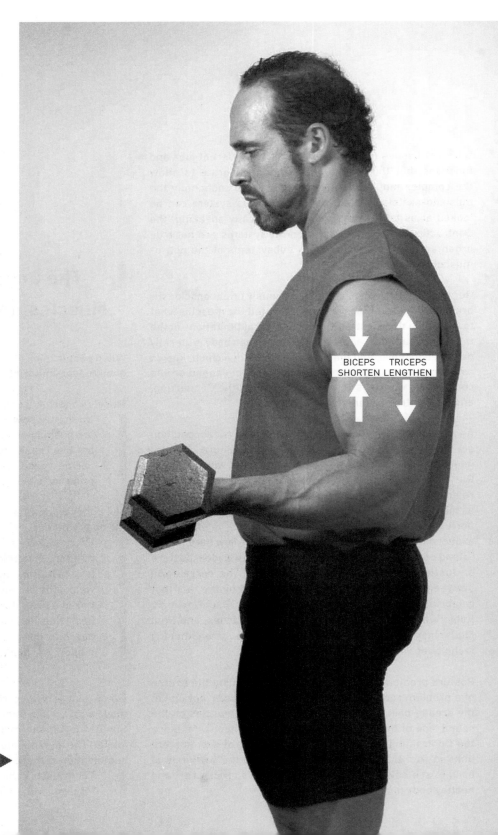

Figure 3-2 Biceps Curl - biceps against triceps ▶

Muscles only contract a short distance but leverage greatly magnifies how far a bone actually moves. For example, the biceps contracts only three inches for the hand to move two feet.

> **"Give me a lever long enough and a fulcrum on which to place it, and I shall move the world."** Archimedes' principle means that the movement caused by a muscle contracting is greatly magnified.

How do muscles get shorter?

Muscles are composed of hundreds of thousands of muscle cells (also called myofibers or muscle fibers).

> Muscle cells range from microscopic to as large as several inches in length, and from far less than the width of a human hair to the thickness of many hairs. Muscle fibers are bundled together by Connecting system membranes called fascia.

Individual muscle fibers create motion in a specific direction when microscopic threads of protein within the muscle pull themselves together. Threads of protein, called actin and myosin, slide along one another in response to a signal from a Control system nerve.

When we move, nerves tell hundreds (or thousands) of individual muscle cells to shorten. However, at the muscle cell level, muscle contraction is an all-or-none affair. Each individual muscle cell is EITHER

> Contracting fully as hard as it can to get as short as it can OR
> It doesn't contract at all.

Known as the ALL or NONE principle of muscle contraction, it's like the digital 1's and 0's of a computer. Just as my computer stores digital music that my iPod plays by saying "sound here" and "no sound there," muscles create Digital Motion because a myofiber is either working, or it's not.

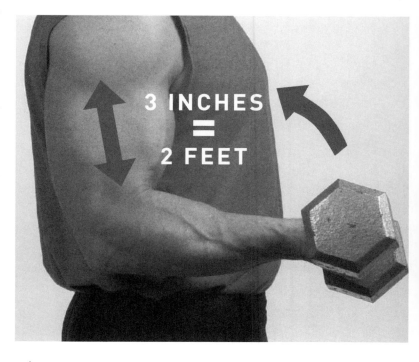

▲ **Figure 3-3** Biceps contracts 3 inches and hand moves 2 feet

46|

»TRY THIS: *Digital Motion demo*

Slowly raise your hand above your head.
Now put it back down,
Lift it again, even slower.

When you lift as slowly as you can, can you lift your hand slowly and smoothly?

If you lift as slowly as possible, most people notice that the hand jumps slightly. You cannot move your hand smoothly and slowly because even though individual muscle fiber contraction is either contracted or not (all-or-none), they work in unison to create the appearance of smooth motion. We perceive motion to be smooth because the breaks in fluid motion happen quickly. A ballet dancer or athlete moves with grace and control because the motion is smooth and well coordinated. This is why an elderly person who cannot control their muscles moves with a jerky walk. Studies show people suffering from chronic low back pain have altered patterns of motion, which means that some muscles contract before they should in a motion and others barely contract at all.

For more information about muscle fibers, including fast vs. slow fibers and more basic anatomy, visit www.bodyzone.com\muscleanatomy.

▼ **Figure 3-4** Digital Motion

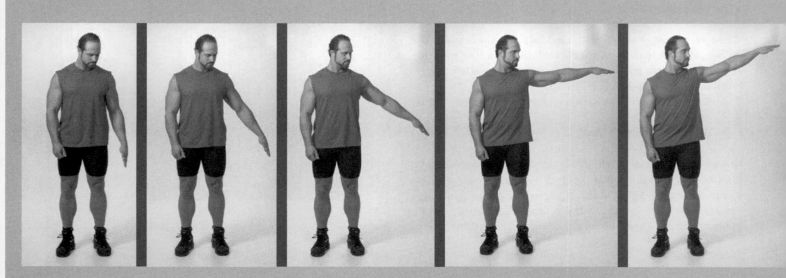

The Dance of Muscle Motion

When you dance with someone, sometimes you step forward as they step back, and then you step back as they step forward. Similarly, muscles work together with their antagonist, or opposing muscle. One pulls as the other lengthens, or both hold steady to stabilize as other muscles take center stage for a particular arc of motion. In a dance of stupefying complexity, we are literally continually juggling flexibility and tightness, stability and motion, in everything we do. While some people look to improve flexibility (a good thing) many people lose sight of the need to constantly stabilize one joint to effectively use another.

In addition to muscles that create motion, there are also sensor muscles. Sensors signal the Controlling spinal cord and/or brain when they are stretched.

> Position sensors can tell the brain the exact angle of a joint (so a golfer knows the difference when she straightens her elbow ever so slightly), or exactly how much stress there is on a joint (as when a pianist easily feels the difference of a tiny fraction of an ounce required to press the keys to play on a cheap piano versus a concert piano).

Depending upon the motion, an individual muscle can play one of four roles in this dance of motion: Agonist, Antagonist, Stabilizer, or Assistant.

Agonist: The main muscle of a motion.

> Motion is powered by the Agonist, or main muscle. The agonist muscle is doing most of the work to accomplish a motion as individual muscle fibers pull a joint in a direction. These fibers work specifically for a particular motion. Depending on the direction of the contraction, the speed (or rate) of contraction, and force of contraction, different fibers within a muscle will contract.

Antagonist: Opposes the main muscle and works to helps stabilize and control motion.

> Every muscle is paired with another that pulls in the opposite direction of the agonist to stabilize and control motion. For example, when I bend my elbow I

am contracting my bicep (agonist) and lengthening my triceps (antagonist). When I reverse the motion and straighten my elbow, the main muscle (agonist) is the triceps, as the antagonist (bicep) lengthens.

We move with control instead of flopping about because in every direction we move[xxiv], main muscles are always being resisted by antagonist muscles and stabilizing the joints. One reason StrongPosture™ exercises are effective at helping back and posture problems is that they teach people new patterns of motion and train unused muscles to work effectively and stabilize motion.

Stabilizers: Keeping it all steady

> *"Stability is the ability to provide support,"*
> Kendal and Kendal, widely used clinical textbook[xxv]

In addition to the stabilization of antagonistic muscles, other "silent majority" muscles known as stabilizers work to provide a firm platform and steady the other movable links.
When you bend your arm to lift a gallon of milk, your bicep is the main muscle, or agonist, but the shoulder muscles have to keep the shoulder still, the neck muscles need to keep your head level so you can see where you are pouring, and your leg muscles have to keep you standing up and balanced.

Assistant (synergist): Helper Muscles

> Synergists are helper muscles that lend a hand to accomplish a motion.
> My small forearm muscles will normally contract when I bend my elbow, but they are not essential for this motion.

CONTRACTING SYSTEM SUMMARY: All muscle contraction does not create motion. Depending upon the motion, a muscle can be the main muscle or a stabilizing opposer, assister, or a stabilizer.

48|

»TRY THIS: *Make a fist*

Keep your right hand open and hold your right wrist with your left hand. Pull your right hand toward you as you resist with your left hand and note how strong you feel.

NOW, repeat with a closed right hand.
Most people notice they are significantly stronger when making a fist.

Why this works: When you make a fist you are contracting the forearm flexors, which are synergists with the biceps.

▼ **Figure 3-5** Open-handed vs. closed-handed bicep curl

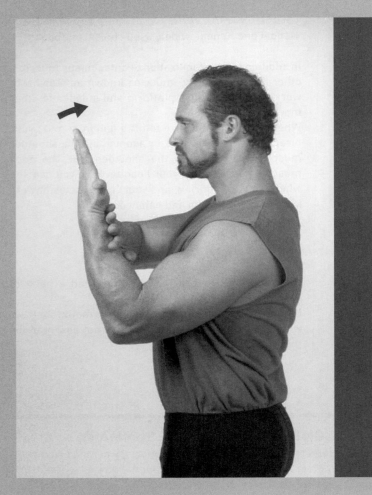
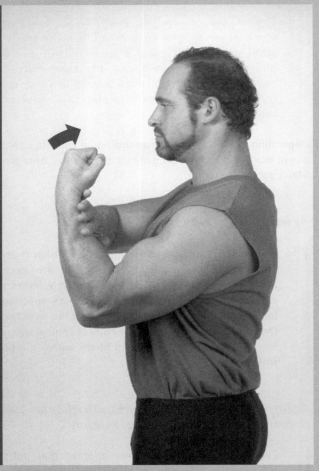

The Connecting System: Holding It All Together

If the muscles of the Contracting system are the motor, the Connecting system is the frame and the tires. Also known as the passive system, the Connecting system consists of everything else holding us together.

The bones are the struts of the body's framework, which are held together at joints by ligaments, which restrain and limit their motion. Cartilage protects bones at the stress points of joints where the bones move. Tendons are the ropes connecting the muscles to the bones. And frequently ignored but very important is the fascia holding everything else together.

Fascial membranes are called the packing material of the body because they surround the muscles and bond all of the tissues into the shape of our body. Also, fascia protects vital tissues by separating tendons, nerves, and blood vessels into appropriate compartments. If you ever took apart a chicken leg, the gristle is the ligament, the meat is the muscle, and the thin membranes are the fascia.

As the main mast of a sailboat holds up the sails, the spine supports the head, arms, and legs. However, unlike the mast of a boat, the spine is a flexible chain of 24 vertebrae connecting the head and pelvis.

The spine is especially important because protected within this flexible chain is the spinal cord, the part of the Controlling system connecting our brain with practically everything in the world. Chiropractors have long claimed to be able to affect and promote general health by realigning vertebra and removing blocks to normal nerve function (called subluxations). This explanation of the often miraculous results seen by many patients is controversial in some circles, but I (along with other scientifically oriented chiropractors) have seen dramatic results in patients for which there are few other plausible explanations.

Movement is especially vital for the spine. The cartilage of the spinal discs has no blood supply after about 25 years of age. The movement of the spine compresses and opens the discs, providing nutrition and waste removal. Without motion, the human spine deteriorates, explaining the epidemic of back problems in a society where sitting motionless for hours is

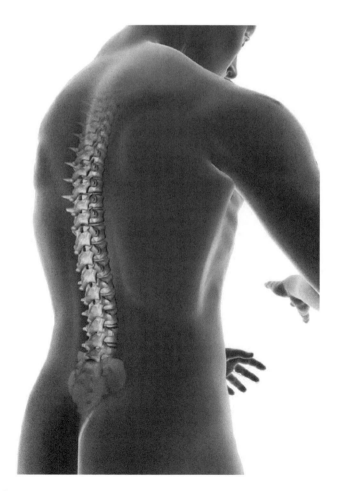

▲ **Figure 3-6** The spine is the main mast of the body

50|

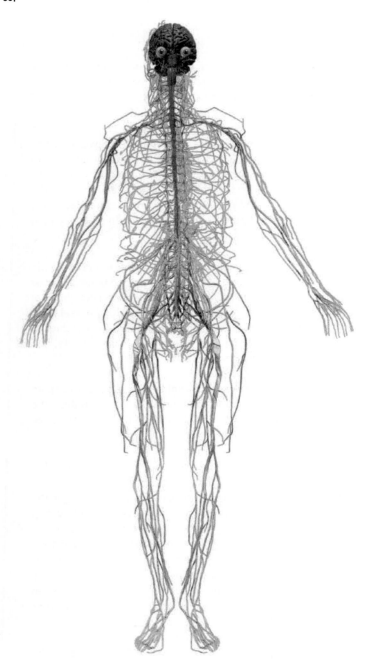

Figure 3-7 Web of nerves -with permission from and copyright of Primal Pictures

the norm. Research shows that with immobilization there is loss of the number of cartilage cells (chondrocytes) within a day, and cartilage substance (proteoglycans) within a week. This is one reason why chiropractors suggest periodic adjustments to keep each spinal vertebra moving and keep the cushioning discs supple.

The Control System
The Central Computer (brain) and Network Cables (spinal cord and nerves)

The Control system tells the body how to move. Nerves tell muscles when to contract, and how hard.

The nerves form a web along which electrical impulses travel to and from the brain via the spinal cord, constantly coordinating how all of the muscles work, and weighing information about tension on muscles, ligaments, and tendons, all the while working to keep you upright.

The Control system controls motion both consciously and unconsciously.

> Conscious motion is when I reach my hand out to pick up a full cup of hot coffee.

> Unconscious motion is when I tighten my shoulder muscles in preparation for lifting my arm, as well as the coffee cup, to take a sip.

> And reflexive motion is when I pull my hand away when the hot coffee spills on my hand if I didn't control my hand's motion well.

For more information about how the brain controls motion, **visit www.bodyzone.com\braincontrol**

The Core of Posture

The Contracting, Connecting and Control components of the motion system are integrated together, and they all affect posture. Whether it's walking with a bad ankle or holding your face with toothache pain, any imbalance, injury, or malfunction of any tissue can affect posture. In particular, the deep muscles balancing the torso over the pelvis play a unique role in posture. Known as the **core**, these deep muscles affect how the whole body moves.

The StrongPosture™ exercises you're learning about in this book (as well as time-tested exercise programs such as Pilates and yoga) focus on the importance of the core muscles with good reason. All body motion begins with and is stabilized by the core muscles. Just as a construction crane needs a stable base to be able to lift a girder, your body needs a stable trunk for you to lift your arms or move your legs.

Professionals from chiropractors to orthopedic surgeons, from massage therapists to physical therapists, and athletes from football players to dancers all agree: core strength is essential for health and optimal performance and aging.

You may never have heard of muscles like the transverse abdominus (TrA for short) or multifidus, but these deep abdominal and back muscles are essential for strong and stable posture.

When these deep torso muscles are engaged and working, they form a muscular "corset" that protects the spine from injury. A weak core means poor posture and a weak low back, and will make you age before your time. Your body compensates for weak core strength with adaptive motions, which sets the stage for injuries.

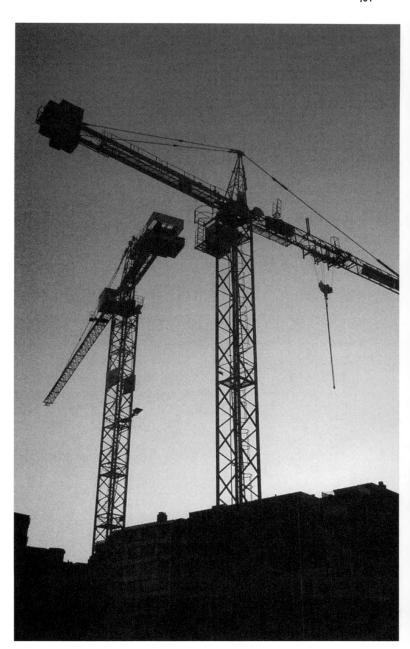

Figure 3-8 Lifting requires a stable base ▶

52|

>>TRY THIS: *Belly-Punch - Tightening the Core*

Imagine someone is about to punch you in the stomach—the belly muscles you reflexively contract are the core muscles of StrongPosture™. They hold everything in like a tuxedo cummerbund.

NOTE: There is an outer set of core muscles[xxvi], but for our purposes, training the deepest inner core muscles is the most effective way to affect posture.

For more on the core visit www.bodyzone.com/coremuscleinfo

The deep core consists of four muscles that wrap around the abdominal organs like a corset.

In front: The transverse abdominus (called the TrA for short)

In back: The multifidus, bracing the vertebra of the spine, our body's main mast.

On the bottom: The pelvic floor

On top: The diaphragm

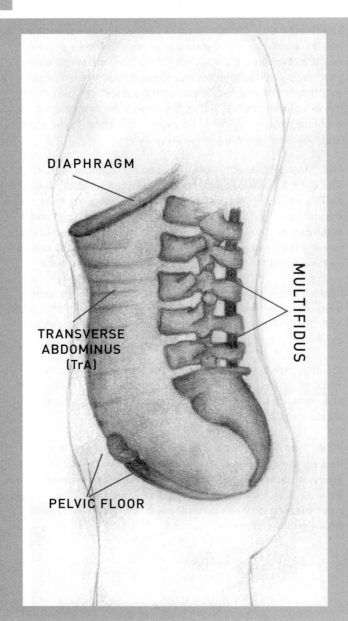

▲ **Figure 3-9** The Inner Core: our postural control system ▶

"Core training" is a hot concept with personal trainers and coaches because strengthening the body as an integrated, holistic unit, rather than isolated parts, is essential for good form. If you want good form in any sport, from golf to tennis, from weightlifting to ballet, strengthening posture and your core muscles makes a tremendous difference in performance. A person with a strong core can run quicker, or hit a golf ball farther or a tennis ball faster, all with potentially greater accuracy. A strong core means a body can stand straighter, look leaner, and be stronger. A stable core means your low back is stable, providing you a stronger base and the ability to compensate for unexpected forces without injury.

TrA- The Core Abdominal Muscle

The deep abdominal muscle is transverse abdominis (TrA) and is an important but frequently neglected core muscle that is difficult to find and train. Despite their hard work doing hundreds of crunches, many people with six-pack abs have weak TrA and significant postural weaknesses.

The TrA lies underneath the rectus abdominis (the six-pack) and its fibers run horizontally so they are not effectively worked by crunches, sit-ups, or other torso flexing exercises. A strong TrA holds in the little "pouch" beneath the belly button that so many people try in vain to reduce. Yoga and Pilates, as well as the StrongPosture™ exercises found in this book like the AbFocus and Superman, teach people to find and use this corset of deep abdominal core and deep spinal muscles.

In the next chapter, you will learn focused, controlled PelvicTilts to find, wake up, and strengthen these unused TrA

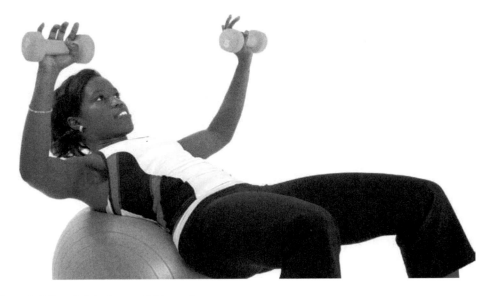

▲ **Figure 3-10** Core Training is essential for performance

deep muscle fibers. One young mother I cared for reported her post-pregnancy belly going away as she went from a size 10 to a size 8 in two weeks after being trained in finding precise control of her pelvic motion, even without the scale budging! Yogis and ballet dancers frequently stay fit well into old age, while many old football players are hobbled with arthritis, bad knees, and stooped posture because of the joint stress from weak TrA and core muscles.

Multifidus

The multifidus are deep back muscles, and are opposing muscles to the abdominals. Multifidus means "many fingers" in Latin, and are tiny fingers of deep muscles connecting adjacent vertebrae. They contract along with other spine extensors, but these muscles are more like sensors (or proprioceptors) that stabilize and support the spine by telling the Control system where and how the torso is moving.

MRIs of patients who have had low back problems show dramatic atrophy of the multifidus, even when the person is not experiencing any symptoms[xxvii]. The reason: regardless of pain, they move in a pattern that avoids these muscles. The solution: training a new pattern of motion. Correctly performed, the pelvic tilts and the Superman StrongPosture™ exercises I will show you are especially effective at targeting this hard-to-find muscle.

Pelvic Floor

The pelvic floor is the "undercarriage" of the body's core muscles. The pelvic floor is a hammock for the internal organs stretching from the pubic bone in front to the tailbone in back, and across the floor of the pelvis.
Weakness of the pelvic floor causes problems holding urine as well as bowel and sexual functions.

For information on strengthening the pelvic floor with Kegel Exercises, visit www.bodyzone.com/kegel

Diaphragm

The diaphragm is the top of the core, internally separating your chest and lungs from your abdominal organs. This sheet of muscle controls breathing, and can dramatically affect posture.

Breathing and StrongPosture™ Exercise

We hold our breath when frightened or when we thread a needle, and breathe quickly when excited, and will continue doing so for as long as there is a breath in our body. Most people breathe without a second thought, but how you breathe not only affects your posture but your mood as well. A deep, full inhale can take in six times as much oxygen as a shallow breath and calm you down, focus, and re-energize as well as increasing oxygen intake to fight free radicals and nourish every aspect of your body. Breathing exercises reduce stress and increase overall breathing capacity.

- ■ Yoga marries focused breathing with exercise, teaching that breath is the door between the mind and the body.

- ■ Psychologists teach stress control breathing exercises for sound physiological reasons, so when someone is emotional or distressed, the advice "take a deep breath" makes sense.

- ■ Chiropractors coordinate with your breath for easier adjustments.

If you have poor posture, you are breathing poorly: mechanically your belly and chest cannot fully open to take a deep breath. Effective StrongPosture™ exercises require coordinating motion with your breathing and controlling the breath to pace the motions of your StrongPosture™ exercises. So, strengthening posture requires breath control, and that means first becoming conscious of how you breathe.

»TRY THIS: *Find your breath*

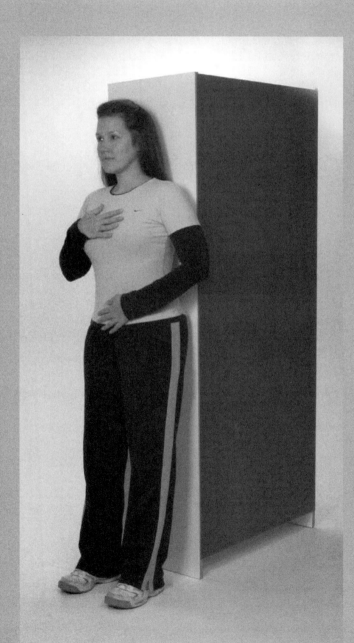

Becoming conscious of how we breathe is the first step in strengthening the diaphragm and breathing.

Stand up and breathe normally, with the waistband loose. (When someone is wearing too-tight pants, they can't breathe diaphragmatically).

Put left hand on your belly

Put your right hand on your chest.

Take 5 slow breaths. Breathe in and out slowly and deeply.

Feel the motion of your left (belly) hand and your right (chest) hand.

If most (**or all!**) of the motion is in the chest, you are a chest breather.

If your belly goes out when you breathe in, and your belly is moving more than your chest, you are a belly breather.

People breathe with their diaphragm, their chest, or some combination of the two.

Diaphragm breathing: Good, strong belly breathing where the stomach goes out when you breathe in, and in when you breathe out.

Chest breathing: Weak, shallow breathing uses the neck, shoulder, and ribcage muscles to lift the chest up, and even pull the stomach in.

Many people are chest breathers, and these people are frequently astounded at what a difference breathing can make. Shallow breathing uses chest and shoulder muscles to elevate the ribcage, resulting in neck and shoulder tension from chronically overworking these muscles (besides giving the body less oxygen). If your neck muscles are lifting your chest with every breath you take, it's not surprising that they will get tight by the end of the day. Over time, all of the body's muscles adapt to your breathing pattern.

Figure 3-11 Find your breath

56|

StrongPosture™ *Alignment:*
Five Breaths Conscious Breathing

Take 5 diaphragmatic breaths, breathing as slowly, as smoothly, as in control as you can. Keep your chest as still as possible.

Breathe **IN** and push your stomach **OUT**

Breathe **OUT** and pull your stomach **IN**

Try to draw in as much breath as you can, pushing your stomach out, hold it for a moment, then

Relax your shoulders, then relax your diaphragm...the exhale will take care of itself.

Repeat, pushing your stomach out and keeping your chest still as you breathe in.

Breathing consciously feels different, de-stressing and relaxing you while giving you more energy. Even though most people can learn to control their breathing with their diaphragm, some people have a difficult time.

Overpressure Breathing (Partner Required)

GOAL: To help chest breathers learn to use their diaphragm.

Start position: As in Find Your Breath, with your right hand on your chest and the left one on belly.

Have a partner put both their hands over your belly hand and press gently.

Breathe in
Push the belly hand out and keep the chest hand quiet.

Breathe out
and relax, letting the pressure from your partner's hand on your belly push the air out.

Partner: Press on the belly as they breathe out.

Breathe in, keeping the chest quiet and pushing against your partner's hand.

Partner: maintain light pressure, but let their stomach push your hand out

Breathe out, pulling your stomach in gently but firmly to force the air out

Partner: Maintain pressure to focus them on breathing with their diaphragm.

Repeat for **5-10** breaths, pressing progressively lighter with each breath so long as the person continues to breathe with the stomach and not the chest.

Many, if not most, people find that when they "catch" themselves breathing during the day, they are chest breathing. Especially if you chest breathe most of the time, taking Five Breaths is a great way to de-stress during the day, and, eventually, you will catch yourself breathing with your belly instead of your chest.

Since the diaphragm controls breathing, it is important to find and use this important core muscle to coordinate your breath with your motion when performing StrongPosture™ exercises. However, people with long-standing habits of chest breathing may find this difficult initially. So, even if you have not completely mastered diaphragmatic breathing, it is important to use your breath to pace your motion while performing StrongPosture™ exercises. In other words, do the best you can, and if you focus on your breath you will find your breath deepening and strengthening as you strengthen your posture.

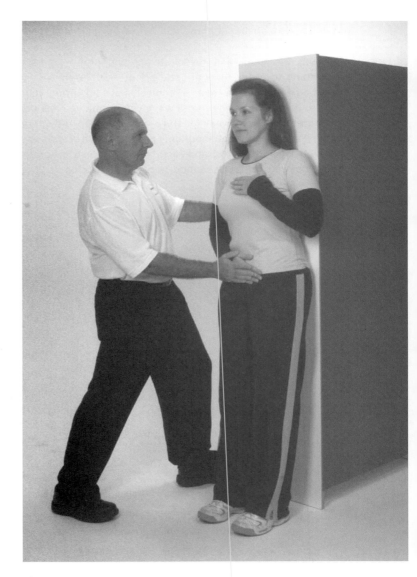

▲ **Figure 3-10** Overpressure breathing

58|

StrongPosture™ Motion: BallMarch–Core Control for Strong Balance

Once you have learned to balance on the ball with StrongPosture™, the BallMarch progression helps you build deep core strength by challenging your ability to stabilize with strong alignment.

Keeping the head and torso strong and stable is very important to train StrongPosture™ in BallMarch. As in One-Leg Balance, the goal is control, not just lifting your leg up. If you dance about and wave your arms you are not strengthening your weak posture muscles. On the other hand, if you are diligent about only progressing as far as you can with strong control and form you'll find you progress quickly as you find and use long-neglected muscles.

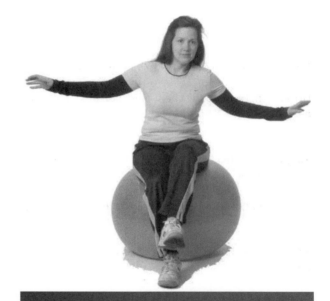

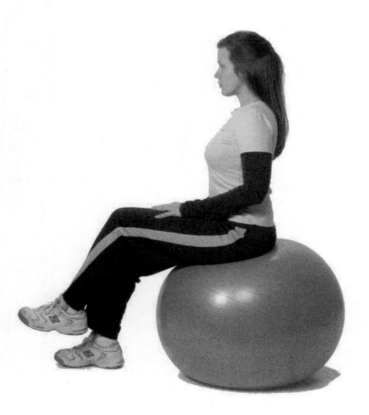

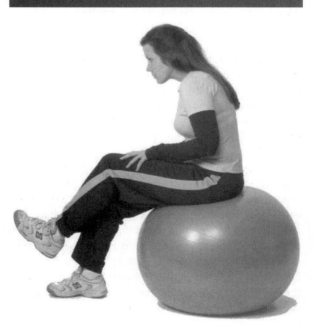

▲ **Figure 3-13** BallMarch with StrongPosture™

▲ **Figure 3-14** BallMarch with weak posture

BallMarch Stability Training A:
BallTilt HeelLift

Start with BallSit StrongPosture™ , feet parallel, and pull your belly in.

Lift your right heel slowly off the ground and put it back down. Keep your posture erect with head, shoulders, and knees strong and aligned.

Repeat with your left heel.

BallMarch Stability Training B:
BallTilt ToeLift

Start with BallSit StrongPosture™ , feet parallel, and pull your belly in.

Lift your right toe slowly off the ground and put it back down. Keep your posture erect with head, shoulders and knees strong and aligned.

Repeat with your left toe.

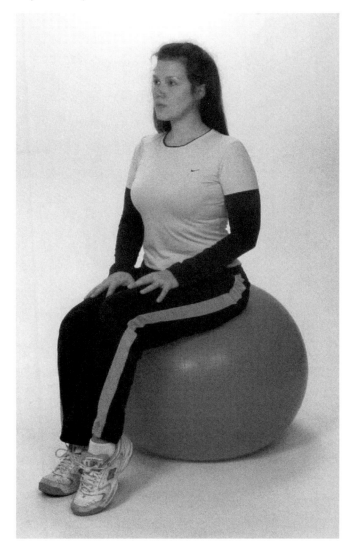

▲ **Figure 3-15** BallSit HeelLift

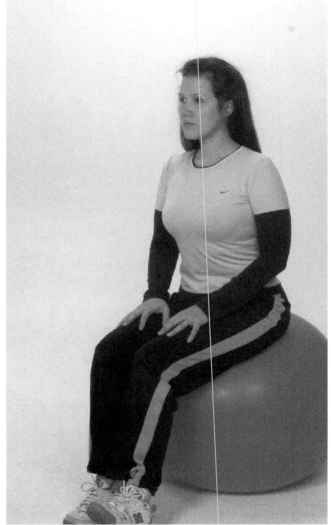

▲ **Figure 3-16** BallSit ToeLift

⁶⁰| *BallMarch*

Start with BallSit StrongPosture™, feet parallel, and pull your belly in.

Lift the entire right foot a few inches off the ground, hold it for a moment, and then put it back down. Keep your posture erect with head, shoulders, and knees strong and aligned.

Repeat with your left foot

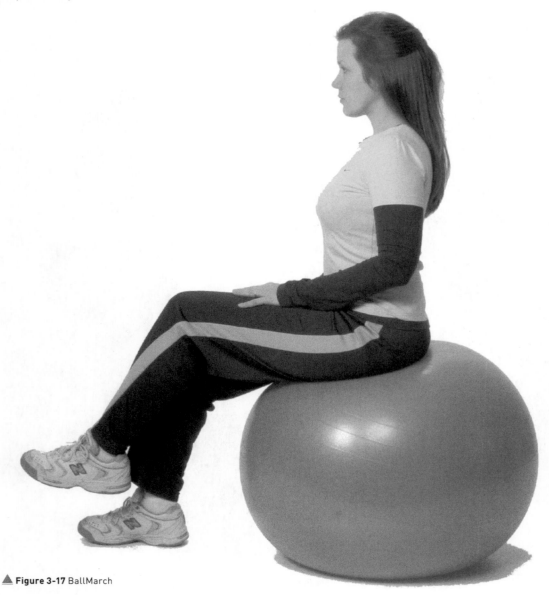

▲ **Figure 3-17** BallMarch

StrongPosture™
7 Week Program-

WEEK 2

B

A

M

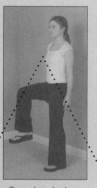

One-leg balance
(**The Stork**)-p.19

Strong Balance

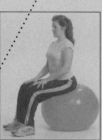

BallSit with
StrongPosture™ -p.34

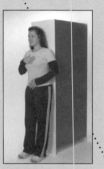

5 Breaths -p55

Strong Alignment

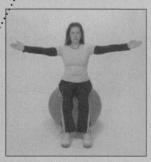

BallSit conscious motion -p.36

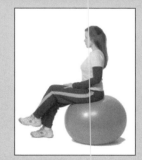

BallMarch-p.60

Strong Motion

3 BALANCE times a day

2 ALIGNMENT times a day

1 MOTION once a day

62|

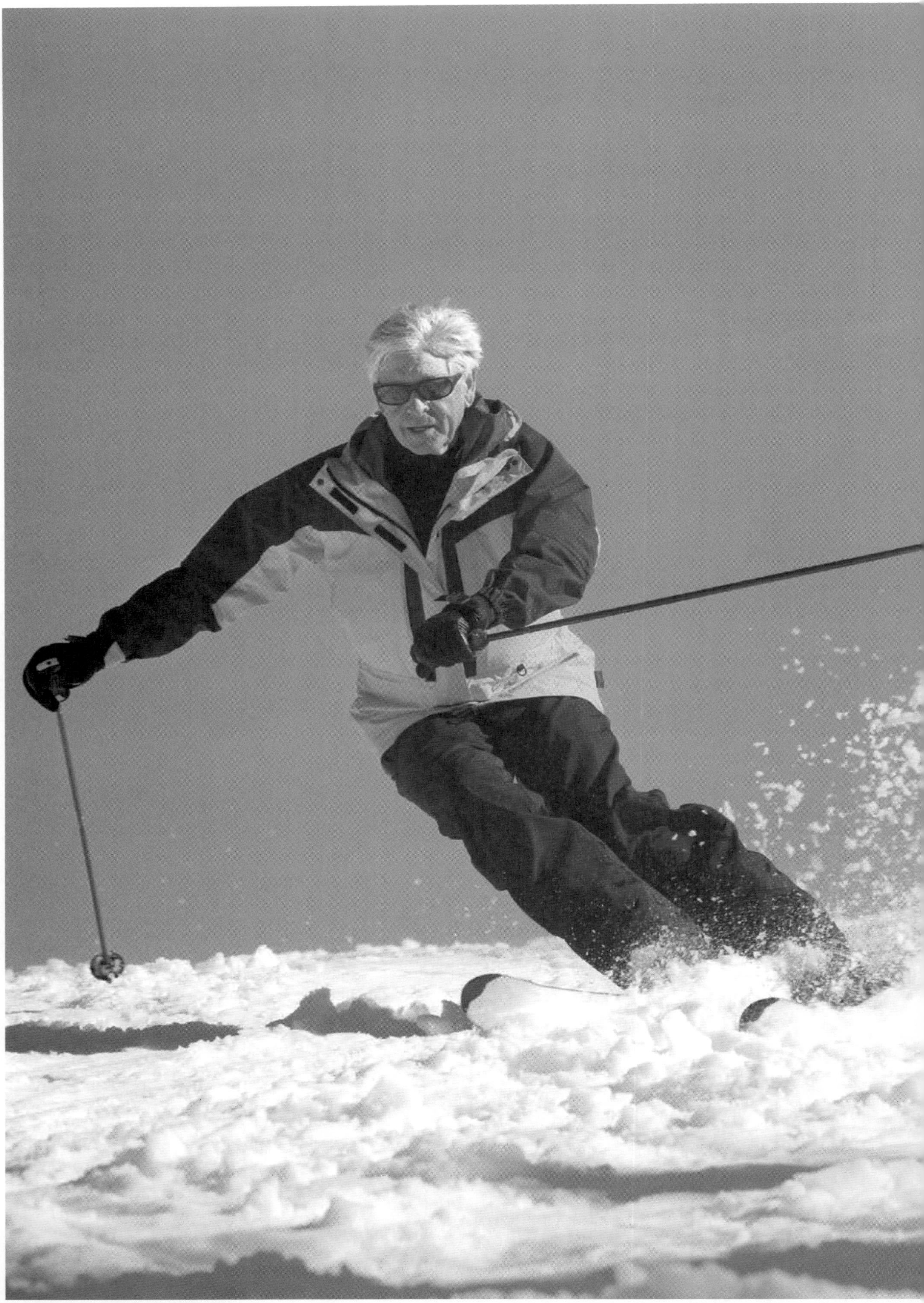

4 Motion
The 1st Posture Principle

The Human Body Is Designed to Move

I am a chiropractor, and I initially looked at the body from the perspectives I learned in school. However, having the privilege of learning from people from other disciplines, professions and adherents of various schools of thought, I am constantly struck by how differently people communicate very similar ideas. Whether someone is a massage therapist, a yoga practitioner, a physical therapist, a personal trainer, a teacher of body motion awareness trained in the ideas put forth by people like Pilates, Feldenkrais, Alexander, or Trager, or a fellow chiropractor, this much I know: All are talking about the same body. The mechanics are the same no matter what: Only the explanations are different.

64 | When people look at the human body they see its incredible complexity through the lens of their own experience. Every field and discipline, from chiropractic to medicine, from massage to physical therapy, and from yoga to Pilates all work with the same human body. There is more to the human body than simple mechanics, but ultimately, the motion of the body is mechanical, and subject to the laws of physics. And everything in the body is connected.

The Five Principles of Posture and Body Motion are a set of concepts to explain the bio-mechanics of how our bodies work. These concepts are universal—no matter how you look at it, anyone who studies how the body moves will agree with these principles. Practitioners of different disciplines may use different words to state it, but I have yet to find anyone who can effectively disagree with these truths. These posture principles are commonsense ideas to help you understand how your body moves, and give you insight into how to keep your body moving well so you can age well.

The first principle of posture and motion is simply this:

The Body Is Designed to Move.

The old saying is "Use it or lose it." It should be "Use it right or lose it," or "Use it to keep it." There is no one single right way to move, but if you let muscles and joints stop moving, over time the overall body loses the ability to move. If you want to move well when you are old, you must keep your body moving well as you age.

Life is motion. When we stop moving, we stop living, which is why staying active is the number one desire of people as they age. When you talk to healthy people over 80, they will almost unanimously say their secret is "keeping active." Motion is vital for health and aging well. Watch a normal child move. Youth is moving freely and with control. Watch someone who's sick move: they are stiff and consequently may be described as "looking old."

Imagine This:

Would you rather stand perfectly still for 30 minutes or walk for 30 minutes?

When we are walking we are doing more work than when we are standing still, so logically you might say standing still is easier. However, almost everyone will agree that it is far easier to walk than to stand perfectly still for a half an hour. The reason moving is easier than being still is that muscles fatigue when they are not allowed to rest. When we walk we alternate between using standing muscles to balance on one leg and shifting muscles to switch to the other leg. This alternation allows one set of muscles to rest while other muscles are working. When we are standing still, we are constantly using the left and right side standing muscles. Even though the amount of work done by each muscle is less, the lack of rest makes the muscle fatigue far more quickly.

Our bodies and our muscles work best when they are worked, and then allowed to rest. When muscles are not rested they become tight, resulting in the chronic "tension" which plagues people who don't move their body. When opposing muscles on both sides of a joint are under equal and constant tension, the joint is not moving. And conversely, if a joint is not moving, there must be constant tension across that joint (usually provided by tight muscles) to keep the joint stable.

Your body has a need to move. If you are typing at a computer for an hour, when you stand up your first instinct is to stretch. When people undergo surgery, they are now required to get up and move around as soon as possible (even though they don't want to). Studies show people heal much better when you get them moving. When you think about it, exercise in general is simply moving your body. It's been said if you could put the benefits of exercise in a pill, it would be the best selling pill of all time. Problems from diabetes to depression, from arthritis to high blood pressure respond to simply getting out and moving your body.

In addition to the obvious muscular and cardiovascular benefits of moving, motion and physical activity pump vital fluids within the body. Cells and tissues with little direct circulation receive nutrition and have their waste products removed by the physical compression and stretching that occurs with motion and exercise. For example, the discs between the vertebrae of the spine have no blood supply in adults, and receive all of their nourishment, including oxygen, from fluid being pulled into and pushed out by bodily motion. When a portion of the spine is not moving properly, the alternating compression and opening of the disc that provides for the exchange of fluids does not occur. Nutrition doesn't get in, waste products accumulate, and breakdown occurs over time. Many experts believe this is why spinal manipulation can slow and even reverse the effects of degenerative disc disease.

There is a neutral range where a body can move, and an accustomed one where it habitually moves. Since muscle function is specific to the way a muscle is moving a joint, part of stabilization training is working muscles (and moving joints) in a full, controlled range of motion to train strength at every angle of a joint's range of motion. StrongPosture™ helps minimize joint and spinal stress, thereby decreasing the risk of injury while maximizing strength and the efficiency of each movement.

Good health requires the ability to move, with control, all the individual links of the body's chain of motion (aka kinetic chain). So the corollary to the first posture principle is:

You must keep moving as you age to keep moving as you age.

The Problem with Sitting: You are not moving

|65

People's bodies are designed to walk and move. Unfortunately, in the 21st century people spend much (if not most) of their lives sitting. We drive to work seated, to sit at a computer, then sit down to lunch, and sit to drive home and sit on the couch and read or watch TV. The result is a body conditioned to sitting. Many people spend the majority of their life sitting with their torso folded and not moving.

Sitting uses some muscles too much and some too little. The overused muscles become too tight, the underused ones too weak, and the joints become stiff from inactivity. Years of inactivity result in the weakening of the body, and balance gets worse. If you don't move your body fully and symmetrically in your daily life, over time things adapt and change. Muscles atrophy, joints stiffen and develop arthritis, discs degenerate, and you become and feel old.

StrongPosture™ exercises train you to move the body with conscious control, in ways you may not usually move, so you can then incorporate previously forgotten motions into your daily life. Adding StrongPosture™ exercise to your regular exercise program is a smart way to keep your body moving well as you age.

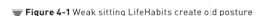
Figure 4-1 Weak sitting LifeHabits create old posture

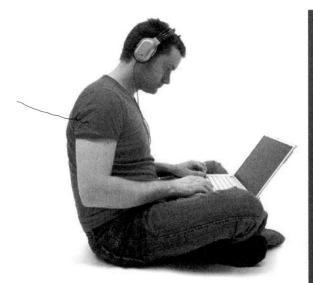

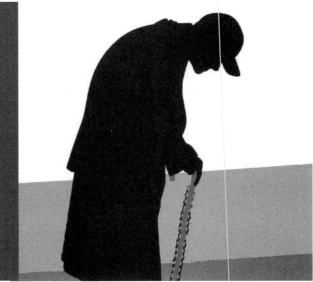

661 StrongPosture™ Alignment:
WallTilts (Focused Pelvic Tilt)

> *"Focused pelvic tilts were a major factor, along with chiropractic, in my recovery from a sacroiliac joint injury."*
> Paula Johnson, First woman to complete the grueling Ironman marathon in less than 10 hours, Canadian Ironman winner, 1988, 1993.

The Focused Pelvic WallTilt is a crucial StrongPosture™ exercise, and creates posture awareness as well as strengthening the core muscles that control posture. Posture patterns exist because we move our bodies in similar patterns, using some muscles more than others. Over time we learn "trick" motions to cheat on good form, giving in to our posture weaknesses.

Like a piano tuner's tuning fork, the WallTilt and other wall StrongPosture™ exercises align your internal perception of where you body is in space with an objective reference, in this case the vertical reality of a wall.

Posture works from the bottom up, so improving posture requires stabilizing the lower body before the upper body. If you try to perform StrongPosture™ exercises for the upper body without first stabilizing the lower body, you will subtly shift your feet, knees, and/or pelvis into familiar patterns instead of moving your upper body in a new, more biomechanically efficient pattern of motion.

Focused WallTilts teach you to move the pelvis and the torso with control to strengthen posture. It's important to master WallTilts before progressing, building a biomechanically stable base from which to progress to other StrongPosture™ exercises.

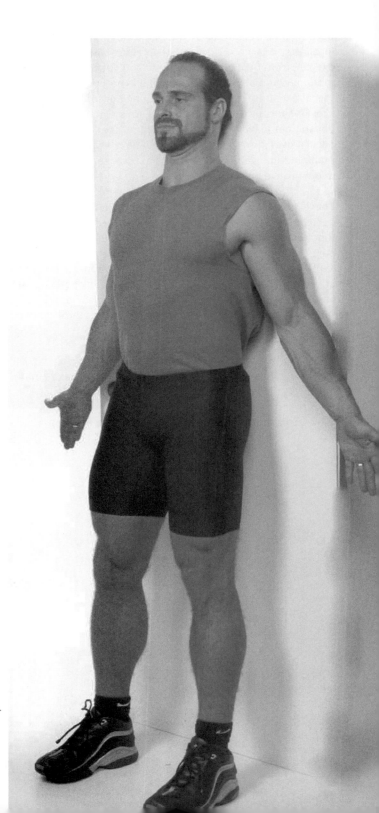

Figure 4-2a WallTilt start position ▶

THE EXERCISE

AWARE POSTION:

Stand leaning against a wall, back straight.

Position feet about a foot from the wall (the length of one of your feet)

> Feet parallel and shoulder-width apart

Knees **LOCKED**, but not hyper-extended.

> Bending the knees to flex the pelvis is a common adaptive pattern of motion. It is far better to move the pelvis only slightly with locked knees than to "cheat" and use a slight knee motion to mimic control of pelvic motion

Buttocks pressed against wall

Shoulders pressed against wall, lowered and relaxed

> Back of hands against the wall, equidistant from the body

> Palms facing forward

Head level!

> **IF POSSIBLE**, put head against wall while comfortably keeping head level, eyes facing forward.

>> However, only go back as far as you can while keeping the head level.

CONSCIOUS MOTION

Flatten your low back so the small of your back touches the wall in a pelvic tuck.

> At the end of your tuck, pull your stomach— especially the lower abdominals—strongly in as you try to press your belly button to the wall.

Then, gently arch your low back in a pelvic arch.

> Move as slowly as you can.

Repeat 5 times, **PRESSING** the tuck, and only **EXPLORING** the arch

BREATHING

The diaphragm is an important core muscle, so when doing WallTilts (or any StrongPosture™ exercise from Yoga to Pilates) it is very important to coordinate breath and motion.

Let your motion follow your breath as you do WallTilts and:

> Breathe **IN**, pushing the stomach out when your pelvis arches, and

> Breathe **OUT**, pulling the stomach in when your pelvis tucks.

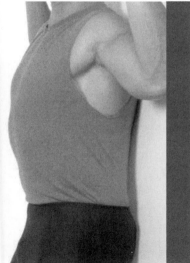

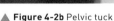 **Figure 4-2b** Pelvic tuck   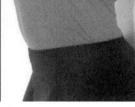 **Figure 4-2c** Pelvic arch

GOAL:

To be able to, with conscious, smooth controlled motion, First tilt the pelvis forward,

> arching the low back into a **PELVIC ARCH**

Then, with controlled motion, flatten the low back,

> tucking the pelvis into a **PELVIC TUCK.**

68| *StrongPosture™ Exercise Form*

Changing patterns requires moving different joints and different muscles. The easiest way to learn a new motion is to focus on only one thing at a time—the problem is, when we move, lots of things are moving. However, if we lock all the links in the body's chain, we can focus on the motion of one link.

Learning to strengthen posture requires fully locking one region, and then moving the targeted region with control. You will be far more successful fully locking whatever needs to be stable 100% (e.g., keeping knees locked), and then working on the region you want to control (e.g., moving the pelvis). If you cheat a little, you're strengthening your old patterns, not building new ones.

So when doing WallTilts, you must keep:

> Knees Locked
> Pelvis pressed to wall
> Shoulders pressed to wall
> Head level
> > Then, if possible, touch the head to the wall.

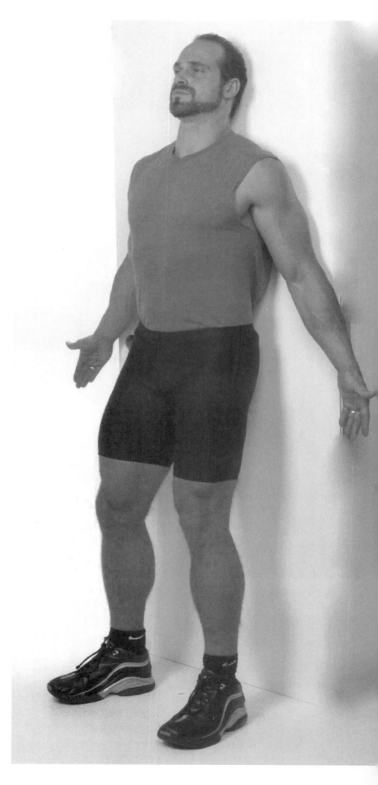

Figure 4-3 Weak WallTilt -Note: Feet point out, ▶
knees flex, head extends and face looks up

FAQ Frequently Asked Questions

Q: How many exercises should I do?
A: Do each exercise for 5 slow, comfortable breaths, letting the motion follow the breath.

Q: How often should I do my StrongPosture™ exercises?
A: I recommend doing Ball StrongMotion exercises once a day and Wall StrongAlignment exercises twice a day (or more if you want a fast stretch and stress reliever). Then do One Leg Balance when you do your other exercises or whenever you think of it. Shoot for spending 30 seconds on each foot, 3 times a day (or whenever you are standing waiting for a minute) to help create a StrongPosture™ LifeHabit.

Q: When should I progress to the next exercises?
A: We usually have patients do pelvic tilts twice daily for 7 days before progressing. This improves pelvic awareness and helps pattern strong, conscious pelvic motion. As you become conscious of your posture and balance, you become more effective at finding new motion patterns.

Q: Are standing pelvic tilts different from the ones I was taught to do lying on my back?
A: Yes! Standing WallTilts require you to balance and support your torso while moving your pelvis to recruit unused muscles. The mechanics of weight-bearing and its effect on the body is also why most chiropractors prefer to take X-rays with the patient standing up. Doing a pelvic tilt on your back is fine for a simple PeelBack, but you want to quickly get to the point of being able to stabilize your pelvis while standing.

Q: Why should I keep my legs away from wall?
A: Bringing the legs away from the wall flexes the torso to change the order of contraction to reprogram which muscles you reflexively use.

WallTilt TrA Focus:

If you are having a problem finding the deep muscles you should be using, try this:

> As you do a pelvic tilt, touch two fingers just inside of your bones on the front of the pelvis.

As you tuck your pelvis, you should feel a muscle tighten. This is the transverse abdominus (TrA). Try to tighten this muscle as hard as you can as you tuck the pelvis, keeping knees straight, head level, and chest relaxed.

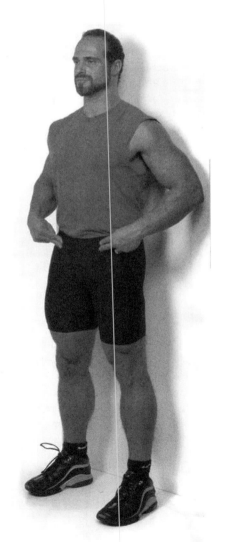

▲ **Figure 4-4** WallTilt Transverse Abdominal (TrA) isolation

701

WallTilt PartnerCheck

A problem with any exercise book or video is maintaining good posture and form. When someone has poor posture and moves improperly, they train the body to continue moving poorly. The WallTilt partner check is a great way to become aware of how your body is truly moving by having a partner review your form. If a partner is not available, go through the following checklist with a mirror.

Spend a few days practicing this new motion and training your muscles, nerves, and ligaments to move in a new pattern so you can train unused muscle and nerve fibers and build a base of strong pelvic motion and control before progressing.

Have your partner read you the following 7 points, Out loud, and One at a time.

> If your form is good, they should say, **"GOOD"** to provide positive feedback.
> If your form is incorrect, they should say, **"TRY TO ...... MORE,"** filling in what you specifically need to modify. When you begin to move correctly, they should simply say, **"GOOD."**

I. Aware Posture Partner Check

As your partner is leaning against a wall, observe their body symmetry. If there is significant side-to-side distortion (e.g., head not over shoulders, shoulders not over hips) suggest they move their _____ a little bit to the left or right, as appropriate. Then read them the following and note their form, from the bottom up, saying **Good** after each observation when they've done it right.

1•Feet should be hip distance apart. **Good**
2•Feet should be about a foot from the wall, squarely and evenly on the floor. **Good**
3•Feet should be parallel, with the heels and toes equidistant and toes pointing forward. **Good**
4•Buttocks should be pressed into the wall. **Good**
5•Knees should be straight and strong, not bent, not hyper-extended. **Good**

> *"Imagine headlights mounted on both knees pointing straight ahead."*

6•Arms should be against the wall, equally spaced from the body, palms facing forward. **Good**
7•Head should be pressed as far to the wall as possible **WHILE KEEPING YOUR HEAD LEVEL**. **Good**

> If the eyes are looking up toward the ceiling, move their head forward until the head is level, eyes facing forward, and then move the head as far back as they can while keeping the head level.

■ A Note About Knees

" You can anger the gods, but never anger your knees."
Bikram Choudhury, famous yogi

You should keep the knees extended and locked but not hyper-extended when doing WallTilts. However, it is important to listen to your body. There is good pain and bad pain. If it hurts, back off. Muscle pain and soreness is usually OK. Straining joints is not. Someone with a history of knee problems or surgery may find doing WallTilts with a small amount of fixed knee flexion preferable to straining the knee back or leaving it unsupported in hyperextension. If knees are an issue, fully lock the knee with the least amount of flexion possible, and then hold both knees symetrically fixed and unmoving while doing WallTilts.

II. Check CONSCIOUS MOTION

The goal is to rotate your tailbone under your body (imagine a puppy putting his tail between his legs).

➔ Try This: Have your partner place a hand behind the small of your back as you push against their hand, pressing to the wall in a tuck.

Have your partner read you the following cues as you do WallTilts:

EXPLORE the arch gently, but **PRESS** the tuck.

Arch your pelvis, sliding your buttocks toward the ceiling.
Tuck your pelvis, push your buttocks to the floor, and flatten your back to the wall.

Arch and push your stomach out like Santa.
Tuck and pull your belly button in toward the wall.

Arch and push your pubic bone toward your feet.
Tuck and pull your pubic bone up and in, toward the ceiling.

Arch, keeping your head level and shoulders and buttocks pressed into the wall.
Tuck and smoothly roll your pelvis under as you extend your spine down.

Continue, checking for good belly breathing.

ARCH
HOLD THE ARCH, and then TAKE A DEEP BREATH IN
TUCK
and BREATHE OUT as you tuck
ARCH
and BREATHE IN while pushing your stomach OUT
TUCK
and exhale while pulling your stomach IN
ARCH
and BREATHE IN, keeping the chest still as the stomach goes OUT
TUCK
and BREATHE OUT, slowly and fully, pulling the belly button into the wall
ARCH
moving with control as you take a deep, slow BREATH IN
TUCK

and slide your buttocks down, pulling your stomach in, and PRESS your back flat as you breathe out

171

Many chest breathers may initially find diaphragmatic belly breathing difficult to coordinate, but this improves with practice and doing the 5 Breaths exercise. Slow, controlled motion with breath control is key to effective focused pelvic tilts. Try to touch every point of your pelvic arc of motion. Moving slowly and consciously, touching every degree of motion, allows you to find and recruit previously unused and forgotten muscle fibers, an important step in achieving pain-free motion with balance, flexibility, and control.

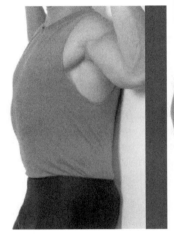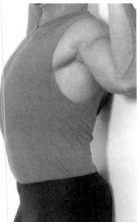

▲ **Figure 4-5** Breath IN on the arch and OUT on the tuck

Also:

■ Imagine writing on the wall with a pen attached to your belt. Move the pen up and down without bending your knees.

■ Imagine a bungee cord pulling your head to the ceiling as you keep your head level, chin tucked and shoulders down. Gently arch your low back as you slowly but firmly tuck your pelvis and pull your lower belly to the wall.

REMEMBER: Firmly Press the Tuck, and Gently Explore the Arch

KEEP KNEES LOCKED and your HEAD LEVEL

PeelBacks and Progressions

72|

The goal is to perform StrongPosture™ exercises perfectly for your body. These exercises are arranged in a logical sequence to teach you to first find and then use your core muscles to control the different motions of the human frame.

If you can't do an exercise perfectly, do a PeelBack (below) that you can do perfectly. PeelBacks are easier modifications of a StrongPosture™ exercise. Be honest with yourself. When you demand perfect form you strengthen your unused muscles and nerve pathways, rather than reinforce bad habits.

On the other hand, if you progress to the point where it is easy to do an exercise mindlessly, then try a progression to further challenge and strengthen posture and balance. Performance-minded athletes find that strengthening balance and posture is a path to improving performance.

PEELBACKS:

If you cannot do a pelvic tilt without bending your knees, lifting your shoulders off the wall, or keeping your head level, try these PeelBacks to help you find and activate your deep core muscles. Do them for a few days, and then try again to progress to a standing pelvic tilt.

If something feels "off" or you feel your form is incorrect even after reviewing the appropriate section and pictures,

consider consulting a BodyZone.com certified Clinical StrongPosture™ exercise Professional (CPEP) to help strengthen your form and alignment.

For more info see www.bodyzone.com/CPEP

Floor Pelvic Tilts

Lie on the floor face up. Let your arms rest at your side and relax your legs on the floor.
Tuck your chin so your head is flat, facing the ceiling.
> If you can't get your head level comfortably, you have a Forward Head Posture. Get as thin of a cushion as you can (folded towels work well) to level your head. When progressing to WallTilts, you will probably find the thickness of the towel will be as far as you should come to the wall while keeping your head level.

Take a deep breath. Note how you feel, and where there is any tightness.
Put your left hand on your belly, beneath your belly button, and your right hand just below your ribcage.
> Arch your back, feeling your hands come apart.
> Tuck your pelvis, pushing your low back to floor, and feel your hands come together.

Feel the abs contracting under your hands. Notice if the upper or lower part of the abdomen is expanding.

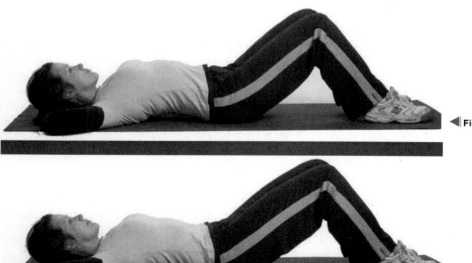

◀| **Figure 4-6a** Floor Pelvic Tilt Arched

◀| **Figure 4-6b** Floor Pelvic Tilt Tucked

PROGRESSIONS:

173

AbSqueeze (Abdominal hollowing)

Once you have the basic pelvic tilt, add a hard abdominal contraction to the end of the motion to fully contract the TrA. When you tuck, at the end of the motion, pull your belly in and pull in the part of your stomach below your belly button. Try to press the belly button as hard as you can toward the spine.

TowelPull Isolation

Hold a rolled-up towel between your thighs by rolling your thighs in and push it toward the wall.
Partner Focus: Have someone apply resistance by gently pulling the rolled-up towel away as you roll your thighs in.

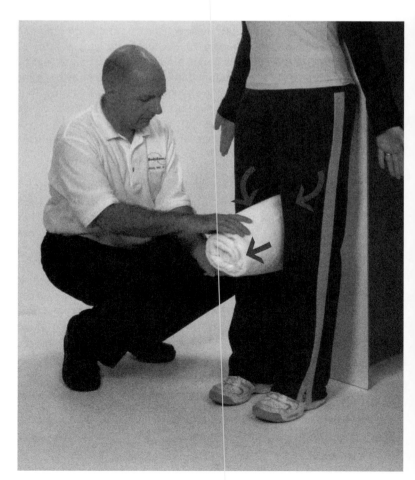

Figure 4-7 WallTilt towel pull

Case History: Pelvic Tilts and Conscious Motion

When we first teach someone conscious StrongPosture™ exercises it never ceases to amaze me how UNconsciously they usually want to move. The key to conscious motion is moving slowly. When we teach someone to do a focused, standing pelvic tilt for the first time, almost invariably they will move quickly. Forcing the muscles to move slower than usual can require considerable conscious effort.

Phillip T. initially presented to us after an auto accident caused soft tissue injuries to his neck and low back. He was a runner, routinely doing ten-mile runs on a weekly basis. Although he had recovered well from his injuries in most of his daily activities, Philip consistently reported low back and sacro-iliac pain after running only four to five miles. He was taught to do basic StrongPosture™ exercises including a pelvic tilt, neck retraction, and beginning ball exercises. When asked to demonstrate pelvic tilts, he tilted and tucked his pelvis smoothly, showing me that he had indeed been practicing them (if someone has not been doing the exercises, it is obvious at first glance). However, I noted that the rhythm of his pelvic tilts was quite fast. After a moment's observation, I realized that Philip was moving his pelvis in the exact same cadence that he used when he was running.

Because his body was trained to move in a running pattern of motion, it was natural for him to do pelvic tilt exercises in his running rhythm. To break this pattern I had him do pelvic tilts at 1/3 speed. It took him a try or two, but once he moved slowly, in the exact same pattern of motion, you could see a light flashing on behind his eyes. When he "got" the motion, he reported feeling his back stretching in a whole different way. Doing the pelvic tilt slowly forced him to be aware, and as a result he felt tight areas in the middle back, which he was not previously aware of, as well as feeling a new stretch in his low back.

Two weeks later Phillip ran twelve miles, pain-free.

StrongPosture™ *Motion:* BallTilt

The purpose of a BallTilt is to train and strengthen conscious, full-range pelvic motion using core muscle control to do a pelvic tilt on the ball.

Independent motion of the pelvis and torso "wakes up" unused fibers in the deep, hard-to-find core posture muscles. Working these opposing core muscles both concentrically (shortening contraction) and eccentrically (lengthening contraction) in a full range of flexion and extension strengthens these often-forgotten muscles.

Before progressing to the BallTilt, you should be able to do a WallTilt.

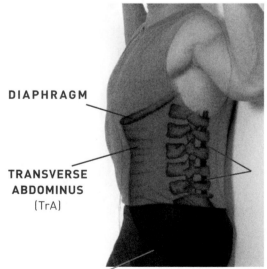

DIAPHRAGM

TRANSVERSE ABDOMINUS (TrA)

MULTIFIDUS

PELVIC FLOOR

▲ **Figure 4-8** Core muscles in Pelvic Tilt

THE EXERCISE

AWARE POSITION:

Sit a bit forward of the top of the ball with the knees at a 90° angle.

Feet should be parallel and flat on the floor.

It is ok to keep your feet wider if you need to, but work to keep heels and toes equally spaced.

Ankles should be aligned directly under the knees.
Thighs level, knees and hips at the same height.
Shoulders over hips.

Roll your shoulders back slightly to lift the chest.

Retract the neck slightly to pull the head over the shoulders.
Hands should be palms up, resting on thighs.

However, if you feel unstable, place the hands on the knees (easier), or on the ball (if necessary).

CONTROLLED MOTION

Move with flowing motion:

Arch your back and slowly, with controlled motion.

The ball should roll back slightly as you arch.

Then, tuck your pelvis into a pelvic tilt
The ball should roll forward slightly as you flatten your back.

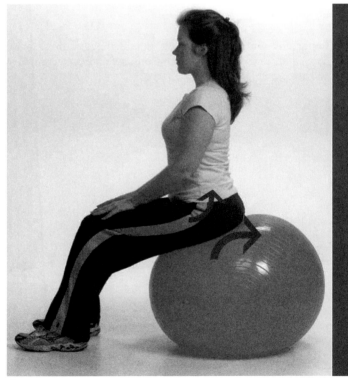

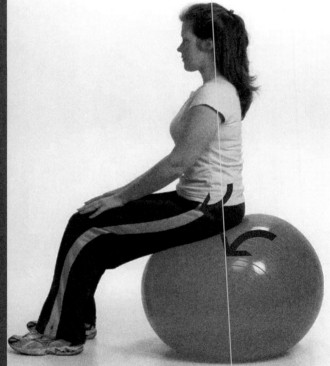

▲ **Figure 4-9** BallTilt Arch

▲ **Figure 4-10** BallTilt Tuck

BREATHING:

Breathe IN as the pelvis arches.
Breathe OUT and pull your belly in as the pelvis tucks.

Breathe in as you arch with StrongPosture™ , neck retracted and sitting tall.

Let your breath drive your motion, breathing as slowly as you comfortably can. Exhale as you flatten your spine, maintaining neck retraction as you pull your belly button toward your spine.
Repeat for 5 slow breaths.

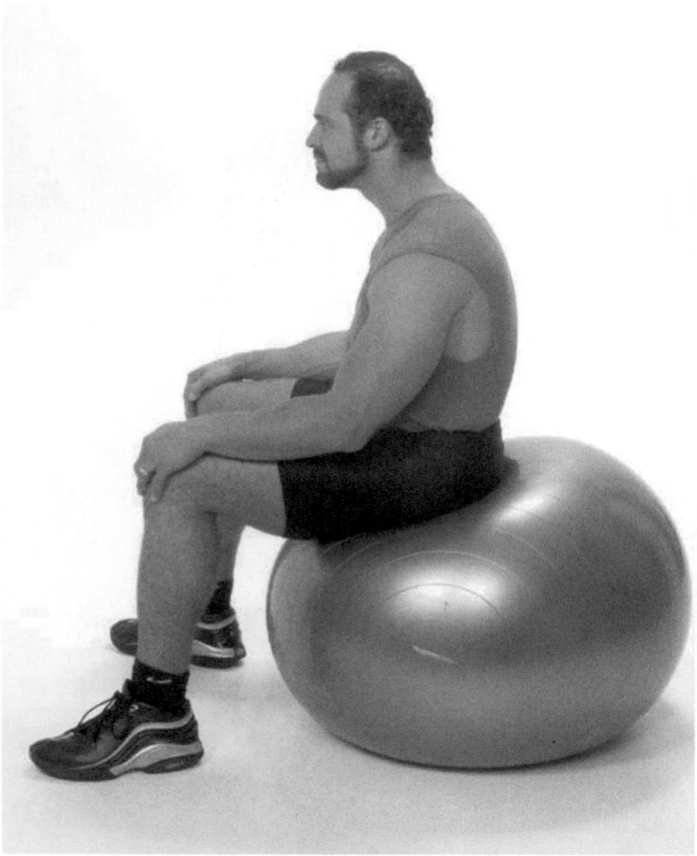

BallTilt Tips

The goal is to **DO YOUR StrongPosture™ exercises PERFECTLY.** Less can be much more when it comes to changing patterns of motion. Performed correctly, a BallTilt isolates the deep core postural muscles and there is minimal overall body movement. The head, shoulders, and knees should be almost still. Also, the ball should move slightly backward when you arch, and slightly forward when you tuck. If you are having a problem doing this, try doing a few WallTilts, and then immediately go back to doing a BallTilt.

PARTNER CHECK:

Have a partner look at you while you do a BallTilt to assess and correct the following.

Aware Posture: Are you sitting up straight, looking forward, and not slumping or leaning to one side? The goal here is StrongPosture™ , so be aware of compensatory motions used to balance, such as slumping or uneven leg placement.

Conscious Motion: The pelvis should move with smooth, slow, and controlled motion; the knees, head, and shoulders are almost still.

▲ **Figure 4-11** BallTilt slump

Many people will not be aware they are moving their knees or shoulders.

As you arch, have your partner put a hand on the front of your knee and say, "Keep your knee against my hand," to help keep you from rocking your knees forward.

As you tuck, the partner should place their other hand just behind your shoulders and say, "Don't touch my hand," to make you aware of when you lean back.

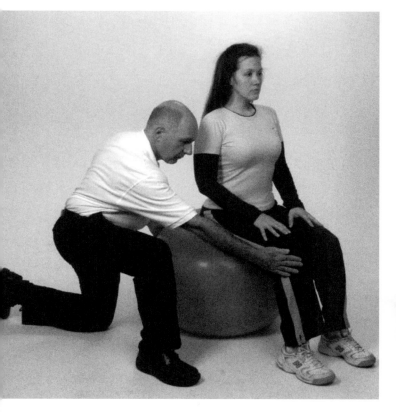

▲ **Figure 4-12** BallTilt partner knee touch

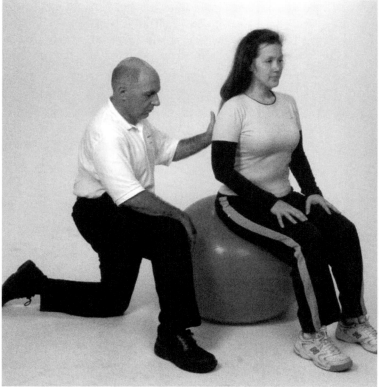

▲ **Figure 4-13** BallTilt partner shoulder touch

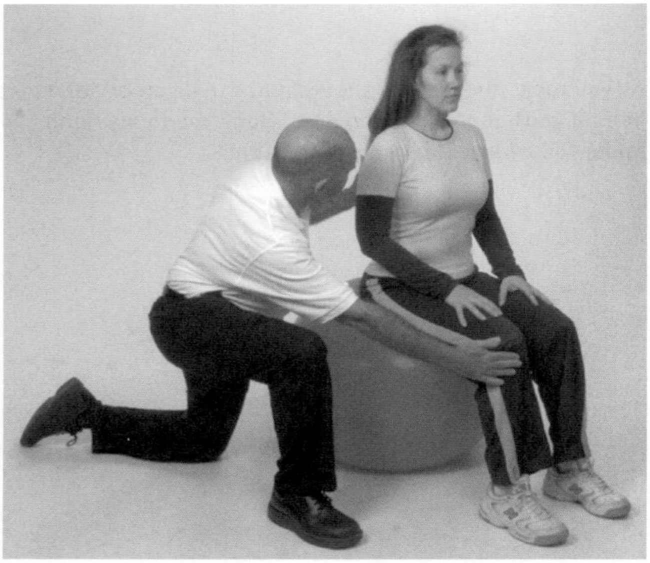

78|

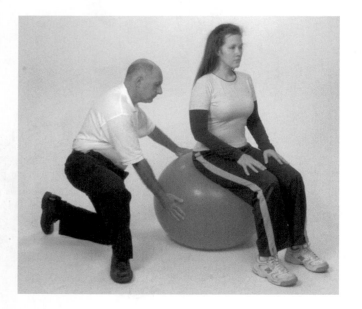

Use your hands to create a "box" within which they do a BallTilt.

By keeping one hand behind the shoulders and one in front of the knees as you do a BallTilt, your partner is creating a BallTilt "box" to help you create awareness of your true body position and use only the deep core muscles to move the ball.

Try to have your partner gently push the ball in the direction it should move when doing a BallTilt to give your brain and muscles feedback on a new motion.

PEELBACKS:

If you are having a problem finding the motion, Be Patient! Usually, the more difficulty people have in isolating the core muscles, the weaker those muscles are and the more they need to strengthen them.

Go back to doing WallTilts for a few days and then try it again, with a partner's help if possible. If you still can't "get it," do the BallMarch (see Chapter 3) for a week, focusing on keeping your belly pulled in.

◀ **Figure 4-14** BallTilt "box"

◀ **Figure 4-15** Assisted BallTilt

B

A

M

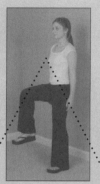

One-leg balance
(**The Stork**)-p.19

Strong Balance

3 BALANCE *times a day*

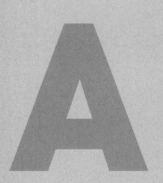

5 Breaths -p55

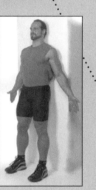

WallTilt -p66

Strong Alignment

2 ALIGNMENT *times a day*

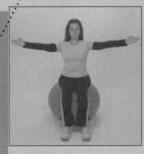

BallSit conscious motion -p.36

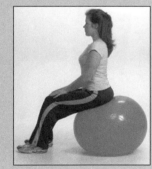

BallTilt Arch -p.75

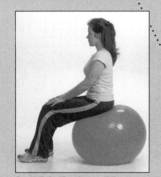

BallTilt Tuck -p.75

Strong Motion

1 MOTION *once a day*

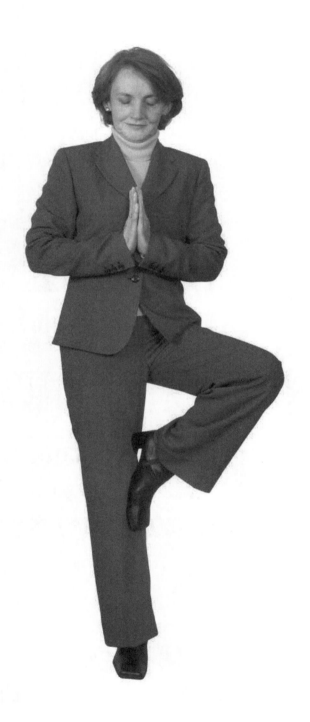

Balance
The 2ⁿᵈ Posture Principle

▌ Posture is How You Balance
Your Body

> *The Riddle of the Sphinx:* What animal walks on 4 legs in the morning, 2 in the afternoon, and 3 in the evening? *ANSWER:* Man. He crawls on all fours in the morning of his life, 2 legs in the afternoon, and with a cane, on 3 legs, in the evening of his life.

The 1st Posture Principle deals with motion. The 2nd Posture Principle is about the other side of the coin: balance.

Think about it: If you don't balance, you fall down! Your posture and your body motion are not symmetrical, but as long as you are not falling down, your body is balanced. If you are standing, your posture may be distorted, and your muscles may be working harder than they should to hold you up, but you are mechanically balanced.

82|

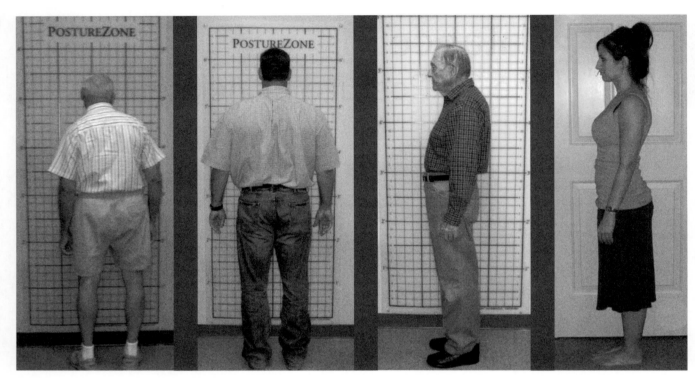

▲ **Figure 5-1** Which of these postures is balanced?

Which of these postures is balanced?

ALL of these postures are balanced. Posture is quite literally how you balance. There are infinite combinations of possible alignments of the joints a body can use to balance. However, there are far more combinations that result in a body falling down. StrongPosture™ is the best biomechanical alignment of the body, where all the muscles and joints are ideally aligned to work their best while stressing the body the least.

The bones and joints of the human frame are NOT very well designed to balance on 2 legs when standing still. Try to stand a child's doll up on 2 legs. If the doll is human-proportioned, it won't be very stable, and it's probably pretty hard to get balanced. If you put the doll on its hands and knees however, it becomes quite stable. Alternatively, adding a cane to a standing doll will make it fairly stable. While someday toymakers may actually sell a geriatric Barbie with a cane, most healthy and active people want to stand on two legs, and therefore must constantly balance their body.

For most of our lives we stand and walk on two legs, balancing effortlessly and unconsciously. We take for granted the amazing ballet of our muscles, joints, nerves, senses, and brain working together in split-second harmony. Walking around takes an astounding amount of information processing to constantly monitor and react to changing data streaming from all over the body, and coordinate muscle activity so you stay upright and balanced. Watch a toddler just learning to walk. The child will stand teetering to and fro, with legs far apart, creating a wide base upon which to balance. After a few weeks of trying, falling, and trying again, the muscles of the Contracting system strengthen and the nerves and reflex pathways of the Control system learn. Balance improves, and the legs come closer together, as the child learns to walk. It's not just the muscles learning, or the brain; the entire motion system adapts and works to maintain balance.

We only think about our balance and how we move when injuries or biomechanical breakdown (arthritis, back pain, etc.) prevent us from moving normally. The man with low back pain learns to walk "crooked" (and thus far less effectively) to keep from hurting, and the woman with the old whiplash injury learns to "just rest her head." Both are adapting their LifeHabits so they can continue to balance while dealing with pain or adaptations from old injuries. Even when balance deteriorates to the point where using a cane makes it "easier to get around," we are still constantly balancing our body.

»TRY THIS: *Up Against The Wall* (Standing Wall Balance Demo)

Balance is deceptively sensitive: every little shift one way must be compensated by moving something else another way.

Stand straight, with good posture, at 90° to a wall with your left shoulder touching the wall.

Try to lift your right leg.

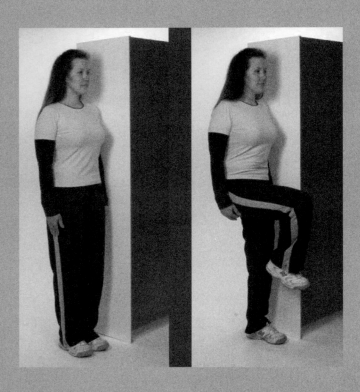

▲ **Figure 5-2** Up against the wall A

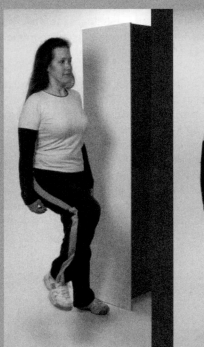
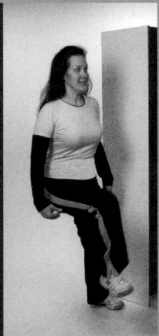

▲ **Figure 5-3** Up against the wall B

Can't? Here's why:

The wall keeps your body from shifting left in order to balance. The shift required is unconscious but real.

The result: you can't lift your leg!

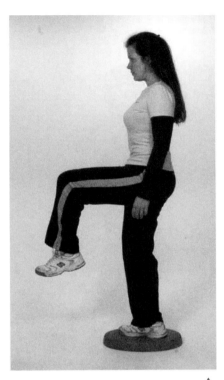

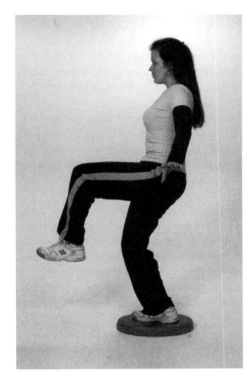

Figure5-4 Strong one-leg balance on balance training pad 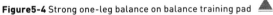 ▲ **Figure 5-5** Weak one-leg balance

When we balance on one leg instead of two, the body has to shift. If the core muscles controlling posture are strong, you can keep the head and shoulders over the pelvis.
If the core is weak, the whole upper body must move to compensate.

StrongPosture™ means that all the muscles and ligaments are able to work their best, with minimal stress, as the body balances.

It is not only the weight-bearing joints (that is, the feet, ankles, knees, hips, and spine) that affect posture. To a greater or lesser degree, all of the joints affect the body's position in space, and so affect posture.

I had a very personal experience once in how posture and balance require all parts of the body the first time I skied down an amateur racecourse.

Being young and invincible, I listened to my friends who advised me to ignore fear and point my skis straight down the mountain as I zigzagged back and forth between the race flags. This worked rather well until halfway down when the tips of my skis crossed, causing me to flip over in the air. With excruciating pain my right shoulder slammed into the snow.

After a few minutes the pain lessened. I got up and was able to stand while holding my arm to my side. With macho bravado, I declined help in continuing down the mountain.

That was a mistake.

I quickly found I could not shift my weight without excruciating shoulder pain. Even when I kept my arm to my side to avoid the pain, I could not shift my body to steer. Even though I could stand, every change in my body's pattern of motion I needed to ski required me to use my injured shoulder. To this day, I clearly remember that very long, very slow, very painful descent.

86 | Balance and the Contracting System

Keeping your balance is unconscious most of the time, but constantly staying upright has very real effects on the Contracting, Connecting and Control motion systems.

The long-term result of the subtle stress on the body from wrong postures was first described in 1969 by Dr. Vladimar Janda. A professor at the St. Charles University in Prague, Dr. Janda studied the effects of modern life and posture on a body designed to walk and run.

Scientists who study body motion (sometimes also called Biomechanics) such as Janda describe walking as a controlled fall. We alternate between standing on one foot, and then shifting to the other foot. This controlled loss and subsequent regaining of balance requires constant shifting of all the links in the chain of posture. As the hand, shoulder, or foot shifts, our centerline of gravity also shifts, causing an inevitable change in overall balance.

Janda attributed the biomechanical problems of our sitting society to subtle shifts in posture resulting from years of progressive adaptation and compensation. He identified two sets of muscles:

> **Postural** (or **Standing**) muscles we use to balance on one leg.
> **Phasic** (or **Shifting**)muscles push us forward to the other leg.

Standing and Shifting muscles work together and in a miracle of coordination choreograph together to balance the body for smooth motion.

> When I take a step with my left foot, I am using my right side Standing muscles to balance on my right foot, and my left side Shifting muscles to pull my left foot forward. By the time my left foot hits the ground, I am using the left side Standing muscles, and my right side Shifting muscles to move my right leg in front of me.
>
> For the purposes of simplicity, we will refer to the leg position (standing or shifting) when discussing these sets of standing and shifting muscles, but understand that the right (and the left) side Standing and Sitting muscles are SETS of 200 or so muscles on both sides of the body. All the right Standing muscles are not on the right and all the left Shifting muscles are not on

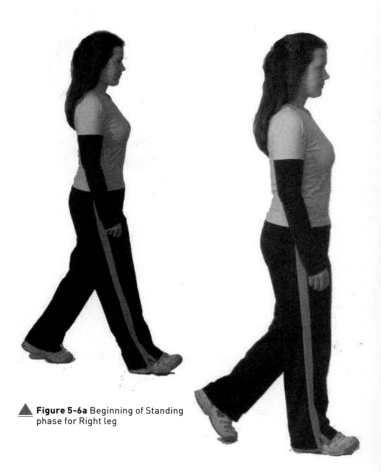

▲ **Figure 5-6a** Beginning of Standing phase for Right leg

▲ **Figure 5-6b** Standing on the Right leg as the left leg shifts forward the left. **See www.BodyZone.com for a summary of the characteristics of standing and shifting muscles**[xxviii].

In order to compensate and balance, the body uses muscles in one of two ways: shifting body position or carrying weight.

Shifting Body Position

We can shift one part forward and something else backward to change our center of gravity.

> The counterbalance for the head going forward is often the chest moving backward. The counterbalance for the chest moving backward is the pelvis tilting forward.

Carrying Weight

We also maintain balance when muscles work harder to hold us up.

> When the head goes forward, the neck and shoulder muscles contract and work harder to keep our chin from hitting our chest. Shoulder tension, neck tightness, and headaches are some problems that occur as frequently used muscles get overly tight, and their underutilized partner muscles weaken.

Weak posture commonly begins with the combination of tight and short standing muscles coupled with weak, overstretched shifting muscles. A pain cycle begins when new injuries occur from the resulting imbalanced motion, creating more compensation from the new injury, which causes the body to further adapt and sets the stage for the next injury, joint wear and tear and ultimately degenerative breakdown.

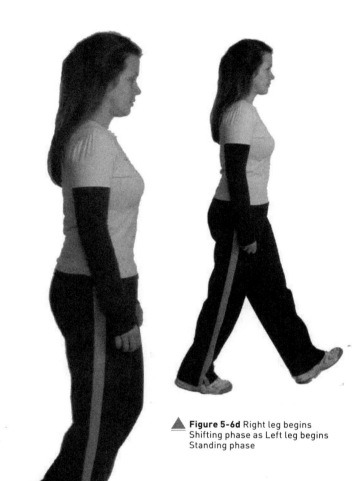

Figure 5-6d Right leg begins Shifting phase as Left leg begins Standing phase

Figure 5-6c All Weight is balanced on Right leg until...

88| Balance and the Connecting System

The bones of the Connecting system form our framework, and are held together at joints by ligaments.

Joints are floppy by themselves, so we contract our muscles to stabilize them as we move each joint through its normal range of motion. We can best control a joint at the middle of its range of motion, where our muscles are working. This "sweet spot" of motion is also called a joint's Neutral Position, and is the best tradeoff of stability and leverage for muscle strength.

StrongPosture™ is the sweet spot for strong balance.

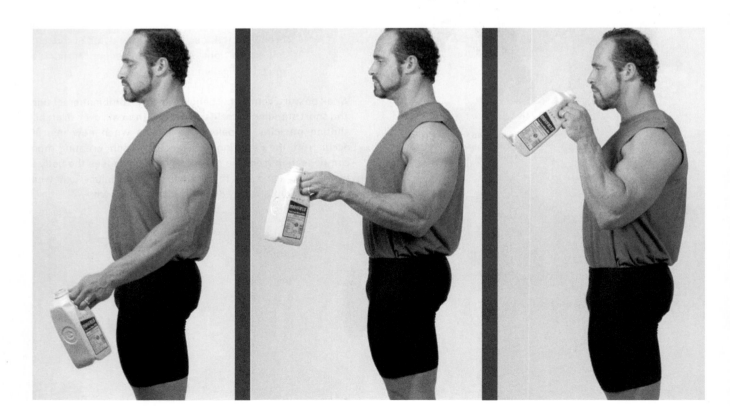

▲ **Figure 5-7** Contracting (shortening) the biceps muscle moves the elbow joint through its range of motion

Balance and the Control System

Balance isn't EITHER-OR...it's AND.

Standing straight and maintaining balance is a surprisingly complex task requiring an incredible amount of Control system activity[xxix]. Not only does the brain learn, but the entire Control system—the brain, spinal cord and the nerves—are constantly working to keep us upright against the pull of gravity and provide a stable platform for our eyes to see and hands to touch and otherwise manipulate our environment[xxx].

In order to balance, our brain integrates information from three major sources to know where our body is in space, and to control it moment by moment as the center of balance shifts with motion. If the input information from the three sources doesn't agree, our balance suffers as the brain tries to find what is level.

Information from these three senses tells the brain where you are in space:

1. **The eyes** (visual sense)
2. **The ears** (vestibular sense)
3. **Muscle and joint position sensors** (kinesthetic sense)

1. The visual sense- our eyes

Vision is the primary source of input to the brain about balance: we see what is level. Motion sickness and dizziness occur when the eyes incorrectly think the body is level but the ears, muscles, and joints sense motion. That is why focusing on the horizon rather than looking inside the boat helps seasickness: the eyes can then perceive the motion being sensed by the ears and position receptors.

2. The vestibular sense- our ears

Inside the inner ear are tiny hairs with tiny stones on the ends of each hair. When we move, the stones tend to stay in one place and bend the hair, which is attached to a nerve that senses motion. I have always been amazed at how this tiny organ senses acceleration and constantly sends information to the brain about how the body is moving.

The dizziness of an ear infection results from the nerves of one ear being stimulated and sending

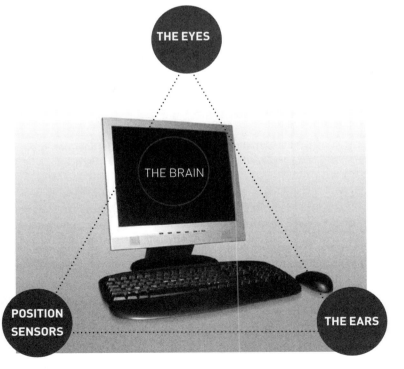

▲ **Figure 5-8** Like a computer, the brain constantly gathers and integrates information about where the body is in space

90|

incorrect information to the brain about how the body is moving. Dizziness is also called vertigo, and can be caused by spinning around in a circle, or riding an amusement park ride, because the fluid in one ear is going in a different direction than the fluid in the other ear, sending conflicting information to the brain.

3. Position - The forgotten sense

Our kinesthetic sense is how you know you are wiggling your fingers or waving your arms even though your eyes are closed. Sensors within muscles, ligaments and tendons (called mechanoreceptors and proprioceptors) are constantly sending the brain signals about position from every joint in the body.

A constant flood of data bombards the brain with information, which the brain processes with split-second precision and sends back out along the nerves to control and coordinate the simultaneous workings of millions of muscle fibers. To maintain balance, the brain and spinal cord constantly receive information about where the body is in space and then tells muscles what to do to keep it balanced.

Mechano-receptors in the feet, hips, and spine are vital to balance and control posture by telling the brain where the body is in space. The brain assumes we are balanced when the sensors report equal stress on both sides of the body.

If the information from these three systems does not agree, we perceive the neurological confusion as dizziness.

> Have you ever gone down a staircase in the darkness and miscounted the number of stairs? That moment of sudden, heart-stopping vertigo you experience is the confusion from the brain expecting the floor to be there when it isn't.

An especially large concentration of these receptors is found between the upper vertebrae of the neck, which is why many vertigo patients have found chiropractic spinal adjustments so helpful.

Balance, Motion, and Pain

People who suffer from chronic low back pain don't move normally[xxxi], and they don't balance normally[xxxii]. Chronic low back pain sufferers have poor balance, even in the absence of current pain, because they cannot rely on information from their proprioceptors and so must rely more on their eyes and ears

> Low back pain patients are usually weak on the one-leg balance test. Also, even though balance exercises with the eyes closed are more difficult in general, patients with a history of low back problems do especially poorly with their eyes closed, even when they are not in any pain.

A key to an effective spinal and StrongPosture™ exercise program is preventing excessive stress in the end-range of joint motion by learning how to more effectively control balance. Training the brain, nerves, and spinal cord of the Control system to teach Contracting muscles to control joints without stressing the Connecting ligaments is essential for effective StrongPosture™ exercises.

To find core muscle control and strengthen balance, try adding some of these BallMarch progressions to the BallTilts you are already doing. Then we'll add BallStretch to your daily StrongPosture™ exercise program.

StrongPosture™ Motion:
BallMarch Progressions -

Challenging Core Control for Strong Balance

If you are ready, here are some Progressions to add to your daily StrongPosture™ exercises.

BallLegLift

1. Start with BallTilt StrongPosture™ , feet parallel, doing a tuck.
2. Lift your right foot slowly off the ground, and then straighten it in front of you and put it back down. Keep your posture erect with head, shoulders, and knees strong and aligned.
3. Repeat with your left foot.

BallLegCross

1. Start with BallTilt StrongPosture™ , feet parallel, doing a tuck.
2. Lift your right foot slowly off the ground and rest it over on your left knee. Keep your posture erect with head, shoulders, and knees strong and aligned. Lean forward if you feel stable.
3. Repeat with your left foot.

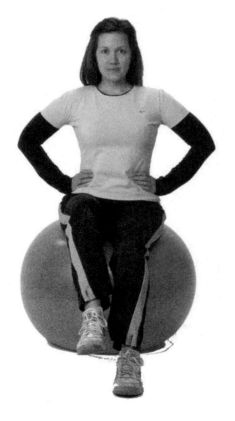

▲ **Figure 5-9** BallSit LegLift

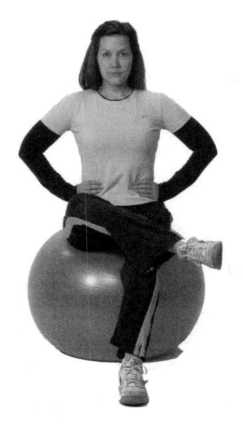

▲ **Figure 5-10** BallSit LegCross

92|

Other BallTilt Variations
ArmsUp BallTilt:

Stabilize your shoulder girdle by keeping your hands on lap, palms up, then pull elbows in, then down.
Then, while maintaining a strong neck posture, lift your arms UP.

By now you have experienced the difference a pelvic tilt makes when stabilizing on a ball, an important step in strengthening posture. Here are a few variations to challenge yourself (or strengthen your specific weakness if recommended by a StrongPosture™ exercise professional). Try them first without, and then while, stabilizing with a BallTilt.

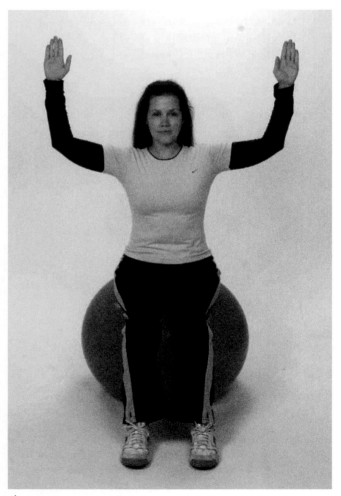

▲ **Figure 5-11** ArmsUP BallTilt

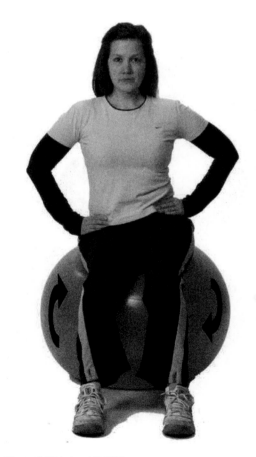

▲ **Figure 5-12** Lateral BallTilts

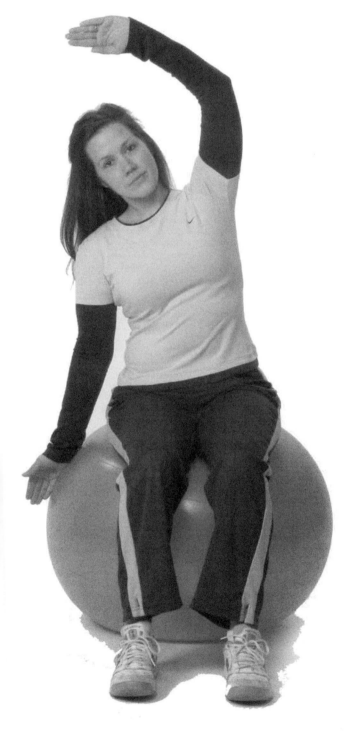

Figure 5-13 Sitting SideStretch

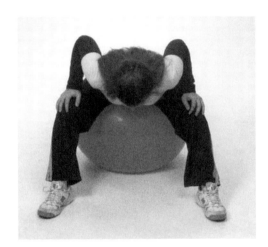

Figure 5-14 Forward Bends

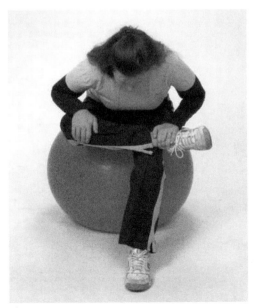

Figure 5-15 CannonBallTilts

StrongPosture™ *Motion:*
BallStretch (aka BackStretch)

94|

BallStretch is the relaxing anti-gravity body stretch to help reverse the folded posture of sitting and wake up unused core muscle fibers.

▼ **Figure 5-16** Sitting spine slump

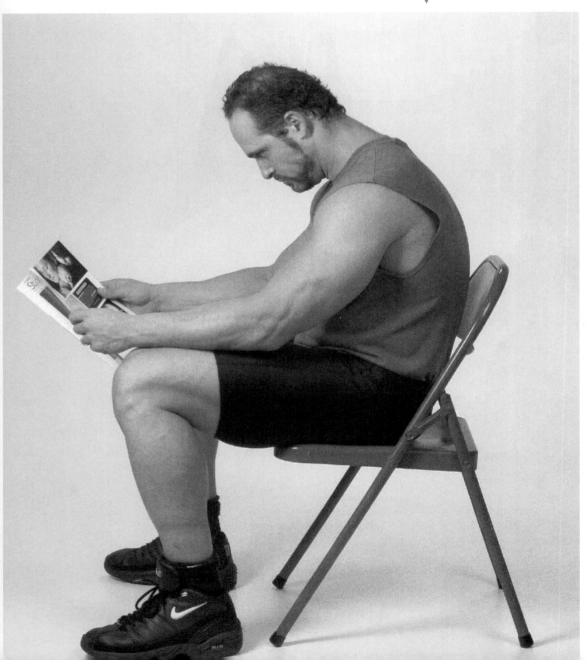

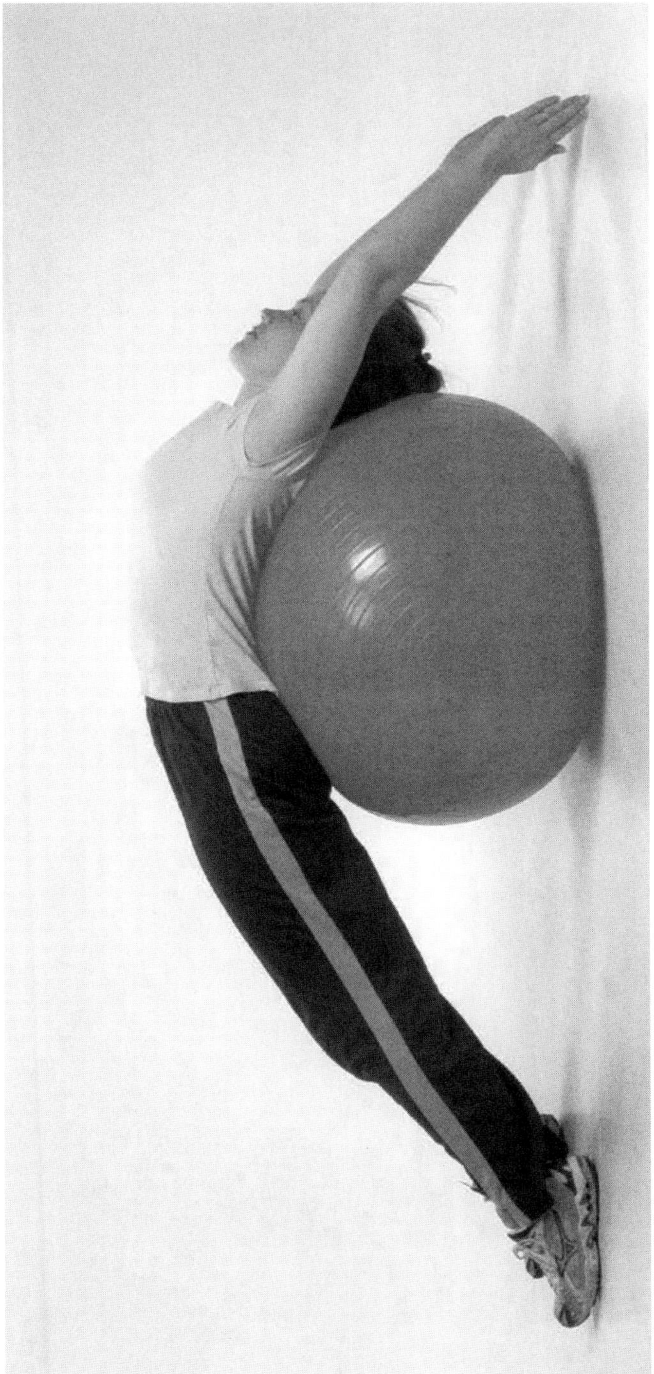

THE EXERCISE

The purpose of the standing pelvic tilt is strong alignment by teaching your body what it feels like to be aligned with something objectively straight, like a wall. The purpose of the BallStretch is training StrongPosture™ by training you to use strong alignment and balance as you move.

Strong Balance + Strong Alignment + Strong Motion = StrongPosture™

BallStretch isn't just flopping around on your back: a strong BallStretch is a controlled flow of motion, a succession of biomechanically coupled motions in the pelvis, spine, and other joints designed to train StrongPosture™ . It's important to tuck your pelvis when moving into, and out of a BallStretch. If you need to use your hands, you are not using your core muscles.

NOTE: We strongly suggest having a partner spot you by standing next to you until you are stable and confident you can balance in BallStretch.

Figure 5-17 BallStretch spine extension

96|

AWARE POSTURE

From BallTilt, begin with a slight pelvic tuck and move
with controlled, flowing motion.
First, walk forward until your head touches the ball
     Bend your knees and let your bottom go toward the floor

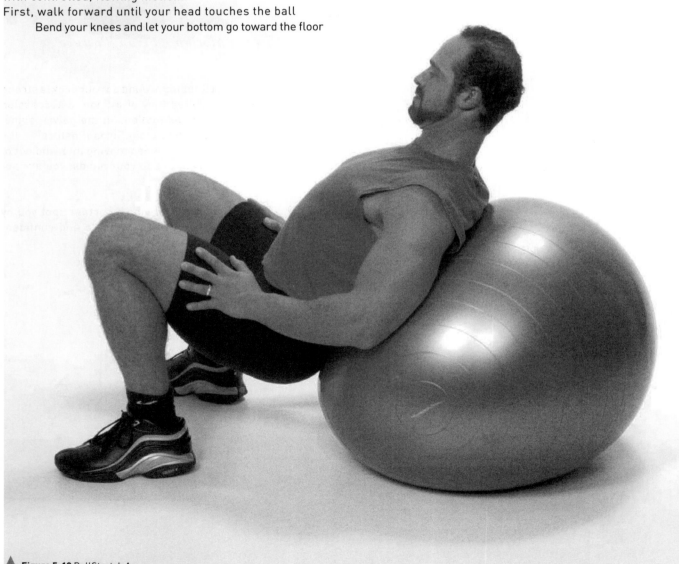

▲ **Figure 5-18** BallStretch A

CONSCIOUS MOTION

IMPORTANT: Keep your head on the ball going into, and coming out of, a BallStretch.

Slowly push your head backward and allow your spine to curve and lengthen over the ball.

Keep your neck slightly retracted and relax your pelvic tuck as necessary. When you feel stable, reach your arms overhead and try to touch the floor.

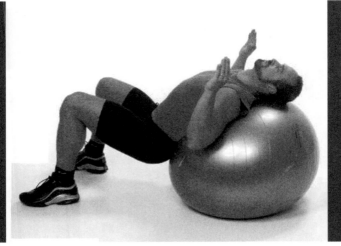

▲ **Figure 5-19** BallStretch B

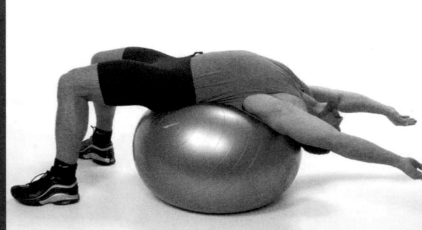

▲ **Figure 5-20** BallStretch C

98|

Only go back on the ball as far as you feel comfortable. Move with controlled motion and maintain control. Touch the floor if you are able to, but above all, KEEP YOUR HEAD ON THE BALL.

Neck strain can result from lifting the head when someone is stretched back on the ball and not properly braced.

REMEMBER:
1. DO NOT STRESS OR STRAIN
2. USE CONTROLLED MOTION
3. KEEP YOUR HEAD ON THE BALL

BREATHING FLOW: Relax and stretch for 5 slow, conscious breaths.

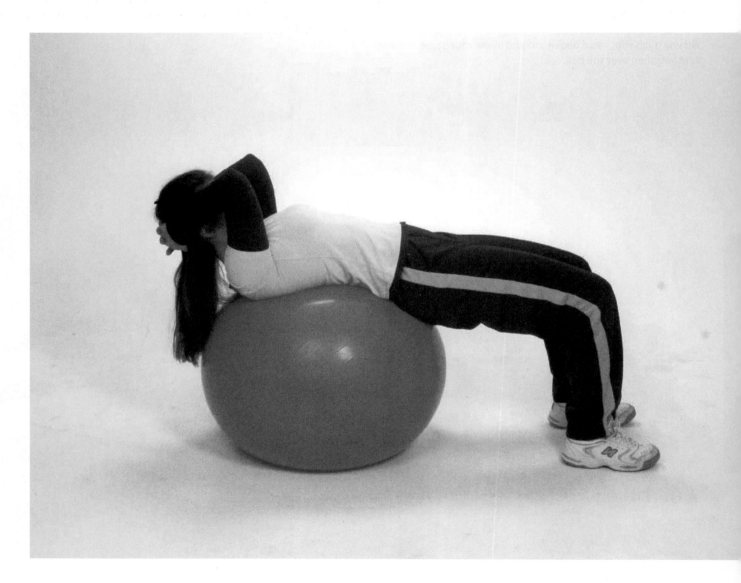

▲ **Figure 5-21** Incorrect BallStretch with head off ball causes strain in neck muscles

Coming out of a BallStretch

1. Tuck your pelvis.
2. Bend your knees and let your seat go toward the floor, keeping your seat and your head on the ball as you lower your hands.
3. Tuck your chin to your chest.
4. Sit up on the ball with core strength by firmly pressing your pelvis into the ball as you walk backward with a strong pelvic tuck.

LifeHabits

The BallStretch is a counter-stretch for the flexed posture of sitting at work.

Ask your boss to OK a ball for break room stretches. Consider sitting on a ball at your desk or put one in your living room to stretch as you TiVo through commercials.

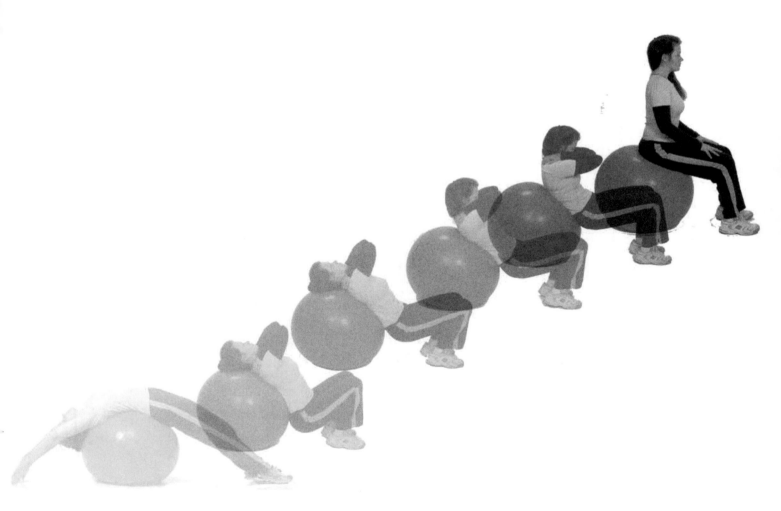

▲ **Figure 5-22** BallStretch SitUP flow

100|

PEELBACKS:

Sit on a padded floor and lean back against a ball. Put your head on the ball and reach back as far as you feel comfortable.

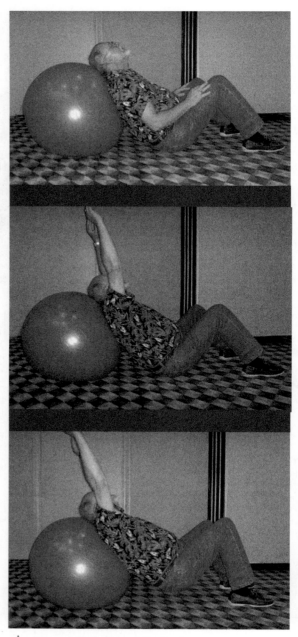

If someone has a severe forward head posture and cannot get their head to rest on the ball, let them try this Peelback

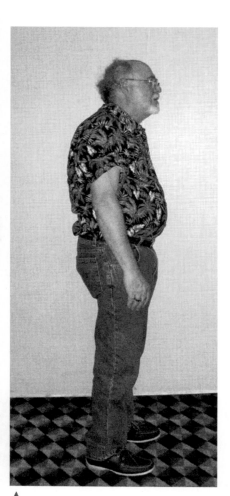

▲ **Figure 5-23a** BallStretch PeelBack

▲ **Figure 5-23b** Severe Forward Head Posture

PROGRESSIONS:

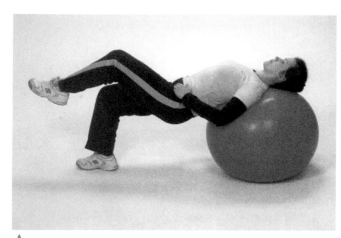

▼ **Figure 5-24** BallBridge

▲ **Figure 5-25** BridgeMarch

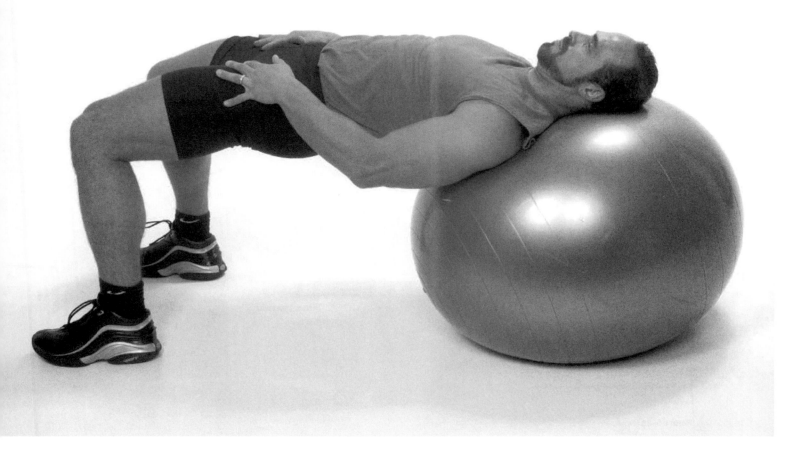

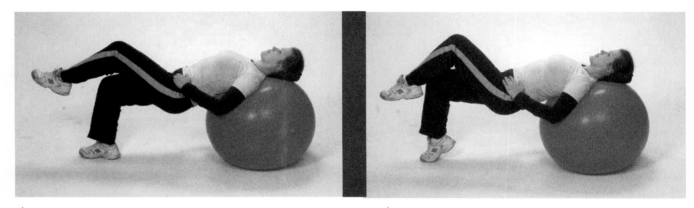

▲ **Figure 5-26** One - leg Bridge   ▲ **Figure 5-27** One - Toe Bridge

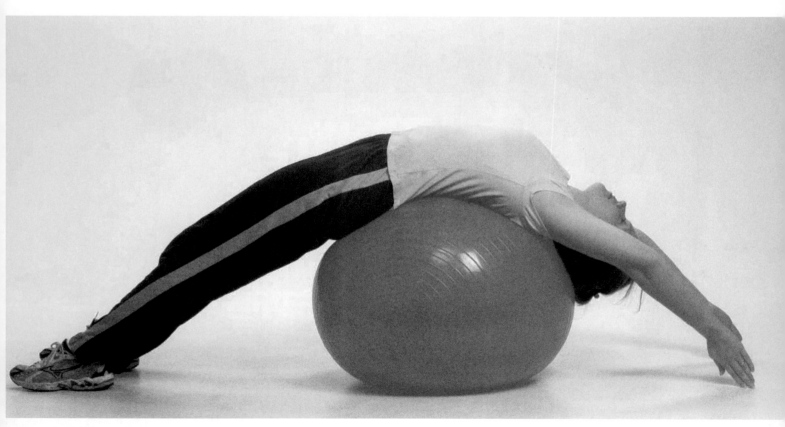

▲ **Figure 5-28** BallArch

StrongPosture™ Motion:
SideStretch
Core Control for Strong Motion

Once you have learned to move the pelvis in a full range of controlled motion with BallTilt and then relax it in BallStretch, the SideStretch progression builds deep core strength by challenging your ability to maintain alignment and balance while moving with control.

Slow motion and strong alignment are essential in SideStretch. Just as a fluorescent light is constantly flickering although it appears to be constantly on, our body motion is composed of thousands of tiny muscle movements choreographed together (see Digital Motion demo). So, to effectively strengthen unused muscle fibers, we need to work joints at frequently unused angles. In building core strength it is imperative to maintain StrongPosture™ alignment *with controlled motion.*

Purpose:

The Ball SideStretch not only opens up the spine and ribcage so you can breathe deeper and move easier, but it can actually help your find where your body truly is in space. Just as posture can feel "right" but a mirror shows postural asymmetry and distortion, the body's motion can feel "right" when we are actually using unbalanced motion.

Balancing in SideStretch aligns our perceptions to where our body truly is—if we are wrong when we think we are symmetrical, we fall. Conscious control of symmetrical lateral torso motion improves balance by strengthening these difficult-to-isolate core muscles and trains the control necessary for strong balance and performance.

GOAL:

Unlock and fully lengthen side spine and ribcage motion with controlled roll over motion. Only go as far as you can with strong control.

> **WARNING:** Skip SideStretch if you have weak balance. We recommend having a partner spot you the first time you try this.

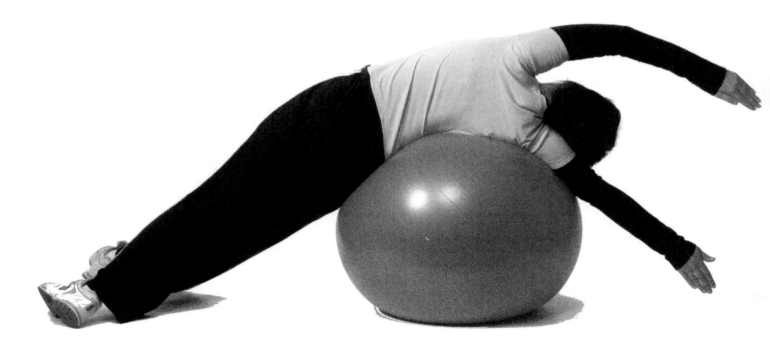

▲ **Figure 5-29** Sidestretch

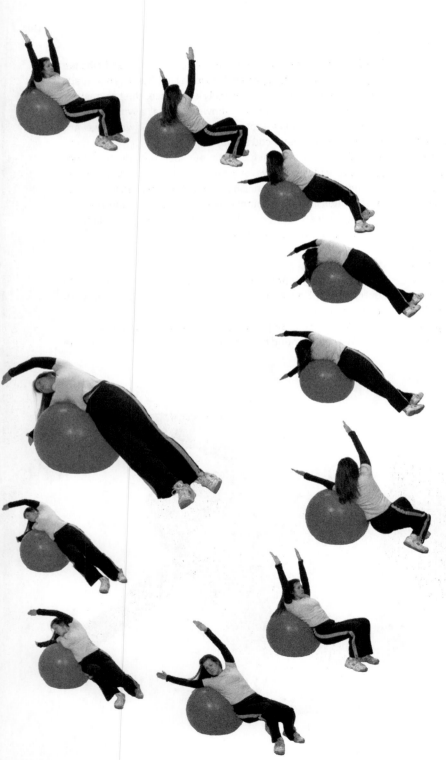

GOING INTO SIDESTRETCH

STEP 1— START POSITION: BALLSTRETCH

STEP 2— DROP AND TUCK

WITH A CORE CONTROLLED PELVIC TUCK DROP DOWN
Keep your head and pelvis on ball as you bend your knees
>   Do not move your feet.
>   Keep hands above shoulders.

STEP 3— Tighten your abs
>   BREATHE OUT AND TUCK PELVIS
>   Use core stomach control
>   Do not move knees or roll ball
>   Pull belly button to spine
Bring chin to chest

STEP 4— Twist
With core control roll onto your right side
>   Keep feet planted- Don't step over

STEP 5—Breathe in as you straighten your knees and reach for the floor
>   Keep bottom edge of feet on floor
>   Keep knees locked
>   Keep hips and shoulders square and head aligned

Hold and relax for two or three controlled breaths.

COMING OUT OF SIDESTRETCH

>   **Bend your knees**
>   **Tuck your pelvis and neck**
>   **Pivot on feet and roll with control**

Repeat on left side.

PEELBACK:
Bend your knees until your buttock is on the ground, then go into a Ball SideStretch from a kneeling position.

PROGRESSION:
SideCrunches (Lateral AbFocus)

 Figure 5-30 SideStrectch flow of motion

StrongPosture™
7 Week Program-

B

A

M

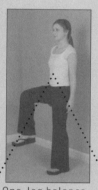

One-leg balance
(**The Stork**)-p.19

Strong Balance

BALANCE

3 times a day

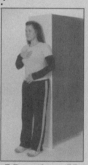

5 Breaths -p55

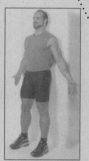

WallTilt -p66

Strong Alignment

ALIGNMENT

2 times a day

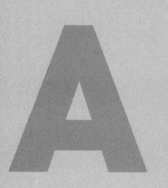

BallTilt Arch -p.75

MOTION

1 once a day

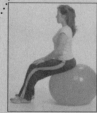

BallTilt Tuck -p.75

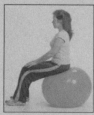

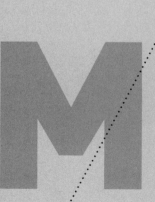

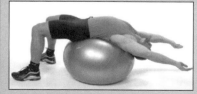

BallStretch -p.96

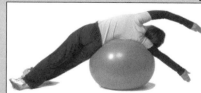

SideStretch -p.103

Strong Motion

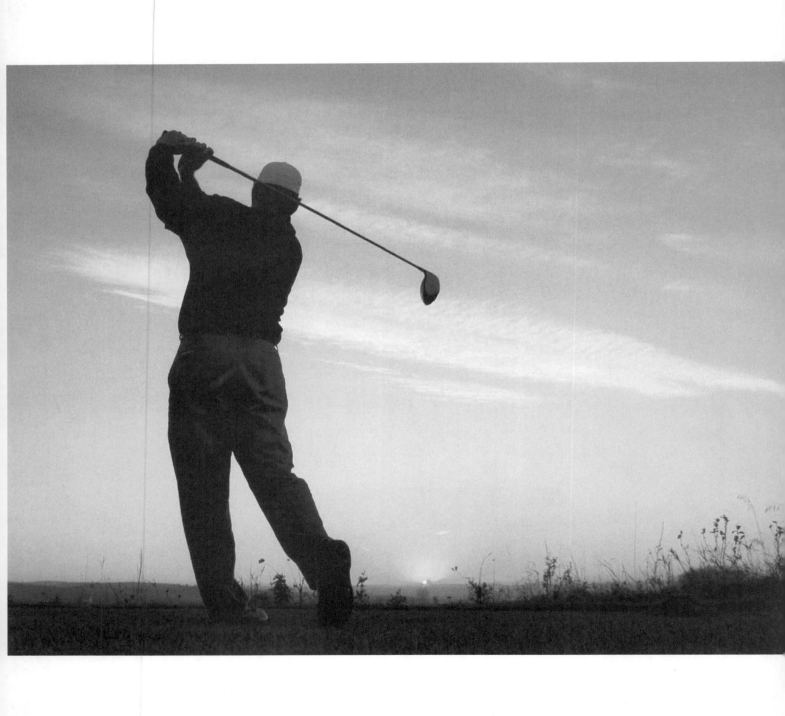

6 Patterns
The 3rd Posture Principle

▌ The Pattern of a Body's Chain of Motion Follows the Path of Least Resistance

> *Following the path of least resistance is what makes rivers and men crooked.* B.J. Palmer, Developer of Chiropractic

The first Posture Principle is about moving our bodies and the second is about how we balance that motion. We live in a delicate balance between mobility–the ability to move–and stability, the ability to resist motion. The 3rd Posture Principle is about the patterns controlling how we move.

In almost everything we do and every motion our bodies make, we move in patterns. All three subsystems of the motion system, Contracting, Connecting, and Control, physically and functionally develop patterns. How we balance the alignment of all the pieces, arms and legs, elbows and knees, head and torso, is a pattern. And in the absence of fo-cused, conscious effort, patterns of alignment guide the body to move as it has before.

Being left- or right-handed is one pattern of motion. Another is which foot you lead with when walking up a flight of stairs. Think about it: do you usually lead with your right or left foot?

Surprisingly, there is little correlation with whether you are right- or left-handed and which foot you lead with. Whether you look at how we pour a glass of milk, lift a heavy box, open a car door, and even in how we sleep, our patterns of motion guide how we move in everyday life. In fact, posture can be de-scribed as the pattern of motion we use to balance our body, standing or sitting.

As I sit here typing, my fingers are moving in complex, coordi-nated patterns using hundreds of different muscles in incred-ibly specific patterns. I am not thinking of how to move my fingers because I was trained to move my fingers in precise patterns on a keyboard to express my thoughts. I learned be-cause of fear of my mom's consequences if I didn't complete my typing lessons, while my kids learned the same skill in or-der to chat with their friends online. In this (as in many things in life), different motivations can result in learning the same patterns of motion.

Motion and posture are holistic, and our patterns of motion are also package deals. As we saw in the 1st Posture Prin-ciple, the contraction of an individual muscle fiber is an all-or-none affair. We are either using a muscle fiber fully, or we are not using it at all. So, when people want to accomplish a specific goal, be it lifting a coffee cup or hitting a golf ball, we use specific muscle fibers in complex combinations that form specific patterns of motion.

Think of the difference between running and walking: when you want to go faster, your gait pattern changes from a walk to a run. A run is not just a faster walk—the motion is qualitative-ly different. And whether walking, jogging, or running, keeping the body in motion requires us to balance our bodies.

These patterns are sometimes called muscle memory, and the learning of these patterns weaves together the Control, Connect-ing, and Contracting systems to create the grooves of motion in which we live our lives. This is why learning a skill is awkward at first, but becomes more familiar with practice. Even if you have

not ridden a bicycle in 30 years, you don't forget how, even if the muscles are no longer conditioned to do it well.

> *"The body thinks in terms of whole motions, not individual muscles[xxxiii]"*
> Irwin Korr, PhD, noted biomechanical researcher

When I reach to pick up a cup of coffee, I don't think about which muscles I am using, or how I am aligning and mov-ing which joints. If I injure my elbow playing tennis and can't properly extend it, I will still reach for my coffee cup, but I will move differently and change my alignment to balance. I won't think about which muscles I need to use more and which ones less to balance and control as I move differently. I just uncon-sciously and automatically move in a way that feels right and doesn't cause pain.

An important technique in clinically studying disorders of posture and motion is simply observing the uncon-scious motion of each muscle and joint, and how it con-tributes to the intended result of the motion.

»TRY THIS: *Don't Be Cross* (Reverse Arm Cross)

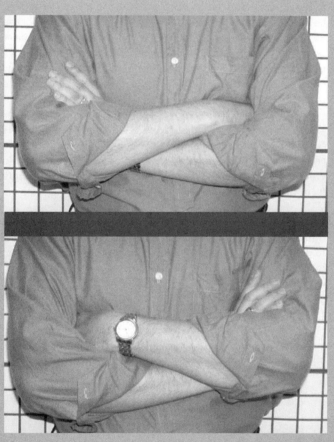

1- Cross your arms.

2- Observe:
  Is your left or right forearm on top?

3- Now, cross your arms with the opposite forearm on top. (Be sure you have a different arm on top this time!)

Crossing the arms "backward" feels awkward to most people. An individual's pattern of motion means they will hold either their left or the right forearm on top. Reversing the top forearm makes the arms, shoulder girdle, and neck move differently from the body's trained patterns. As a very general rule of thumb, the more locked in a pattern of motion (and therefore out of balance) a person is, the more imbalanced they feel on doing a Reverse ArmCross. Some people are so fixed in their pattern of motion they are unable to cross their arms backward without assistance!

"Don't Be Cross" demonstrates that the body moves in patterns of motion, and communicates that chronic muscle and joint problems begin when the body learns to move in a distorted pattern.

Figure 6-1 Don't Be Cross

Figure 6-2 Reverse Thumb Cross

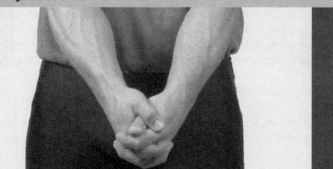

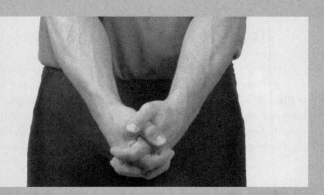

110| ## The Body Moves in a Chain of Motion...

...Your foot bone connected to your ankle bone,
Your ankle bone connected to your leg bone,
Your leg bone connected to your knee bone...
Dem Bones, children's rhyme, author unknown

Our body's motion and posture depend on an interdependent chain of muscles, bones, and joints subject to the laws of physics. Bones go where muscles put them, but they stay where muscles, ligaments, and fascia keep them. Muscles move bones, which in turn are mechanically connected to other bones in the skeletal chain. Generally speaking, in a kinetic chain there are two ways of controlling motion while maintaining stability: only moving one joint at time, or simultaneously coordinating the motion of every link in the kinetic chain.

The first way controls motion by keeping some parts of the kinetic chain stiff and rigid while others are moving. As an example visualize the one-year-old child tottering back and forth with locked knees as they are just learning to walk. Others are the chronic-back-pain patient moving with characteristically restricted motion and the old person shuffling along, both holding back stiff and moving knees and feet only as much as necessary.

The second, albeit more difficult, way to move and maintain balance is by smoothly coordinating the motion and ever-changing position of each individual part of the kinetic chain. Scientists call this coordination and control "coupled motion," athletes call it good form, but the rest of us know it by a more old-fashioned name: grace.

Coupled, Synchronized, Holistic Motion (aka Grace)

Graceful motion is the ideal: smooth, synchronized, and controlled. The 80-year-old woman who looks 45 when you see her walking from behind is moving with grace and StrongPosture™. Smoothly coupled motion is also essential to perform well with good form in any sport. In fact, exercise in general

is more effective when performed with good form (which begins with good posture).

We move our bodies with whole motions that begin with our posture. We don't stop and think about the individual muscles and joints we need to use, we just move everything. If a golfer has distorted posture when standing up "straight," before he even moves his club he has a problem! His address position (the starting position for a golf swing) will also have distorted, adaptive posture so even though he thinks he's standing straight, his swing is compensating. Which is why golfers with postural problems feel awkward when learning a balanced swing.

The problem is magnified because people don't do what feels "awkward." When exercising, as in other aspects of life, we repetitively strengthen what is strong and neglect the weak. Weakness of unused muscles and nerve pathways results from this imbalance of habit and motion.

You usually don't think about how you move, but if you do think about it, you think of what you want to do, not about how to do it or which muscles you need to contract. The quality of motion is how well all the different pieces work together.

Patterns of mechanical alignment and control develop from the combined adaptation of Contracting, Connecting, and Control systems

Mechanical Patterns in the Contracting System

Muscle patterns develop in part for the obvious reason: used muscles strengthen and unused muscles atrophy. As we saw in the Digital Motion demo, muscles are made of muscle fibers, and each individual muscle fiber's contraction is an all-or-none affair. Therefore, a muscle gets stronger (or weaker) specifically in the ways it is used. Overall muscle strengthening is specific to the angle, speed, and phase (i.e., lengthening or shortening) of each motion.

Since muscles strengthen in the ways that they are used, if a joint is never moved in a direction, the individual muscle

|111

fibers of the muscles responsible for that motion are never worked, and weaken over time. Even if a person "feels" strong because of other muscle fibers compensating, motion in only a part of a joint's arc of motion results in a weakening of the unused muscle fibers.

People with posture problems are often told they have weak muscles and advised to exercise. But if posture is weak and motion imbalanced then it's difficult to strengthen muscles with symmetry. Altered posture and body mechanics make an exercise intended to work one muscle target the muscle group differently, or target other muscles entirely.

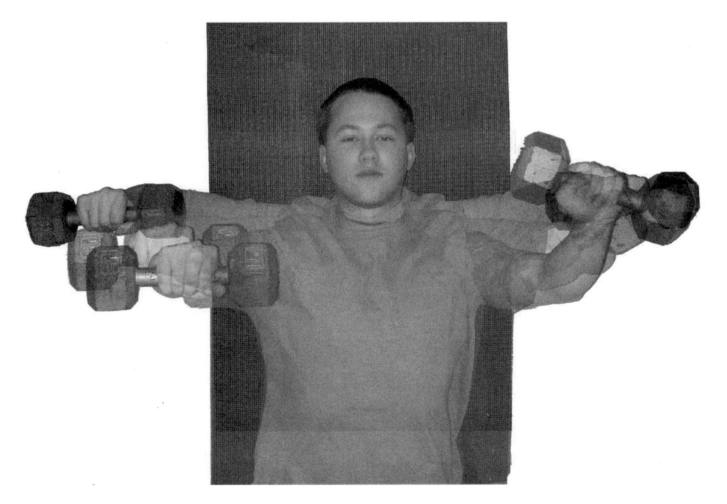

▲ **Figure 6-3** Uneven arc of motion

»TRY THIS: *Milk Jug Curls*

To understand why muscles develop mechanical Contracting system patterns, lift a light weight (such as a gallon of milk) firmly in one hand.

Stand straight with your arm at your side,
Then, bend your arm to 10° and count to 10. Note how hard it is to hold.
Then bend your arm to 90° and count to 10. Is it any easier or harder to hold?
Now bend your arm all the way and count to 10. Is holding it easier or harder?

Keeping the elbow partially flexed and the supporting muscle partially shortened overlaps the fibers, making it easier to hold up the weight.

During normal motion, some muscles lengthen as others shorten. Muscles are strongest and have their greatest holding power when they are fully contracted, with all their fibers overlapped. So, if someone has a problem area, a weak link in the kinetic chain, the easiest way to move is to keep the weakest muscles fully shortened and only move the stronger muscles. In addition, to avoid pain we fully shorten the muscles in the weak area to stabilize by "locking it down", even though this is not necessarily the best or most graceful way to move.

The reason patients suffering with back problems complain of moving "like an old person" is that the injured (and often the elderly) limit motion in weak or injured areas so they have fewer areas to control. Stiff body motion weakens and even atrophies some muscles as their overused partners become overly tight in an adaptive pattern of muscle motion.

Clinical note to posture professionals:
Motion collapses in a kinetic chain of motion at the level of the weak muscles as the weakest muscles fully contract to maintain stability.

Instead of, say, four joints moving 25% to accomplish a motion, a weak link causes a motion "collapse" so other areas take up more motion as the weak areas move less.

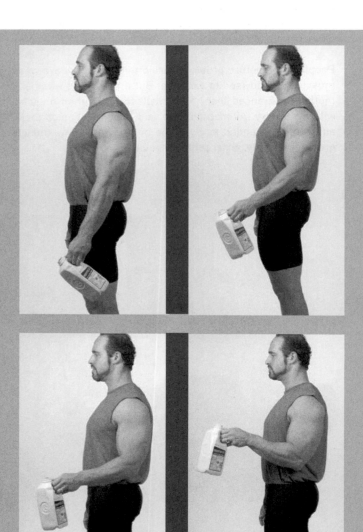

▲ **Figure 6-4** Milk jug curls- Range of motion

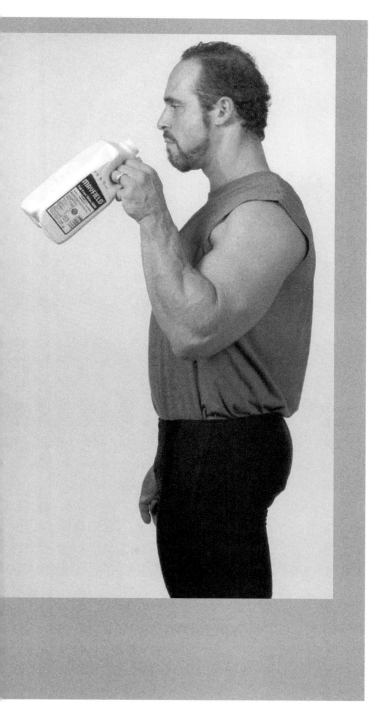

Mechanical Patterns of the Connecting System

Anatomically, the motion of each joint in the chain is limited by the shape of the bones (elbows can't bend backward) and the ligaments holding the joint together, resulting in the anatomical range of motion (RoM). A joint that moves outside these anatomical limits will dislocate, a distinctly painful experience.

Mechanically, patterns develop from the interplay of muscles, and the fibers of ligaments, tendons, and fascia form patterns. Physically, fibers bend along the lines in which the body moves, and lengthen, warp, and shorten, resulting in a functional range of motion (fRoM).

The fRoM is the arc of a joint's motion where the body has adapted to work best. Even though I have met a few gymnasts and yoga practitioners who can touch their heels bending backward, most of us find it is far easier to attempt touching our toes going forward.

However, we spend most of our lives moving our joints in a narrower range called the active range of motion (aRoM), or how far you can move a joint on your own. It is within this aRoM that contracting muscles strengthen and work most effectively, connecting tissues stretch and tighten to guide motion, and nerves become trained to control motion.

One way of looking at the body's motion patterns is to think of a folded piece of paper that, once folded, continues to fold at a crease.

114|

»TRY THIS: *The Folds of Life*

Once creased, always creased.

Take a piece of cardboard or paper and fold it sharply. Try to take out the crease.

You can unfold a piece of paper, but the crease will always remain. You can't ever completely remove the fold because the fibers have been bent in a pattern. Similarly, the microscopic fibers of the Connecting (as well as the Contracting) system change and adapt to moving the body in learned patterns of motion.

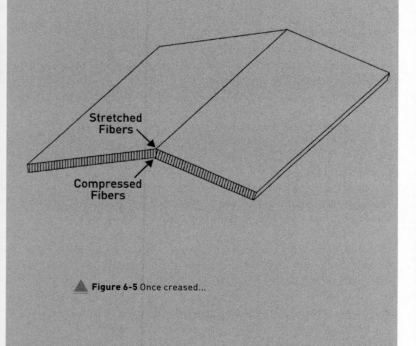

Stretched Fibers

Compressed Fibers

▲ **Figure 6-5** Once creased...

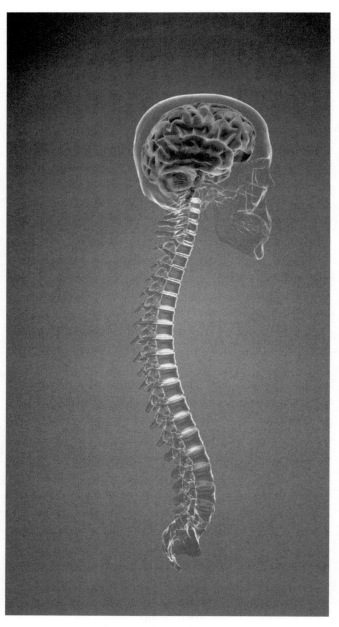

▲ **Figure 6-6** Programs in the brain and nervous system creates patterns of motion

Control Patterns of the Control System

Body motion is a chain, but unlike a metal chain subject to only mechanical forces, neurologic programs of motion ultimately guide our body motion.

Unconscious motion programs in the brain, spinal cord, nerves, and receptors of the Control system work muscles in the ways they've been trained. The more a nerve control pathway is used, the easier it is for the body to use that pathway. The scientific term for nerves getting better at doing what they do is facilitation, but it's more commonly known as muscle memory. Our motion is not only physically controlled by muscles and joints, but by what you have learned to do. The golfer swinging his club, the baseball pitcher throwing a ball, and the little girl skipping rope are all performing complex activities in an incredibly precise symphony controlled by their motion programs.

One reason programming robots to walk is such a difficult technical feat is the astounding coordination and control required to balance a body in motion in even everyday activities. Without thinking about it, our nervous system pools information from all over the body to tell the muscles how to continually adapt to changes in our environment.

»TRY THIS: *Fill'er Up*

Fill a glass with water.

As the glass gets heavier, you automatically adjust your muscular effort to compensate.

Take a glass and, holding it level, fill it with water from a faucet.

Did you have to think about adjusting the force necessary to keep the glass level as the weight of the water changed? Or did you just fill it up without needing to be conscious of, or compensate for, the continually increasing weight of the glass?

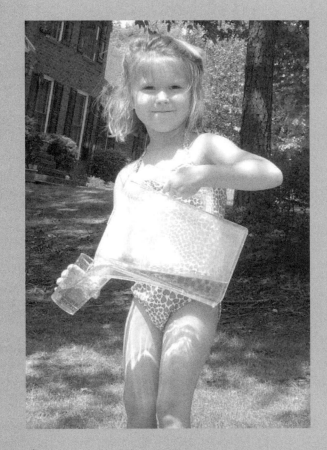

Figure 6-7 As a glass fills and gets heavier (and the pitcher gets lighter) we learn to automatically compensate and avoid spilling the water.

116|

..That Follows the Path of Least Resistance

The architecture of a human body is basically a head with one mouth and two eyes balanced on a torso with two arms balanced on a pelvis with two legs. We are designed to stand up, move forward, look in front of us, and use our hands to manipulate or otherwise affect things in our environment.

Mechanically, posture is how we balance four masses, also known as posture zones. We all balance the head on the torso, which balances on the pelvis, which balances on the legs. Since the motion of each joint is specific in a direction, the result is that people's bodies tend to fold in predictable patterns at three areas where the body naturally "folds":

The pelvis most commonly tilts forward, as the legs, knees. and feet roll in.
The shoulders will most commonly roll forward, as the hands turn in.
The head will most commonly jut forward.

The mechanical stress of balancing follows the kinetic chain of the body's motion along the path of least resistance. As we walk, the foot strikes the floor sending stress up the ankles, to the knees and hips, to the spine, torso, shoulders, and arms, and finally to the head as everything constantly shifts and counterbalances to keep us upright.

Stress always goes to the weakest point in a chain first, where the loose link moves before the stiff link. Mechanically, motion follows the path of least resistance because the most flexible (or least restricted) joint moves first and the least flexible (or tightest) joint moves last. As in any chain, our bones, muscles, and joints move along the path of least resistance. In addition to limiting the overall pattern of motion, the tightest link in a chain is the last to move so it also creates increased stress and abnormal motion in adjacent areas.

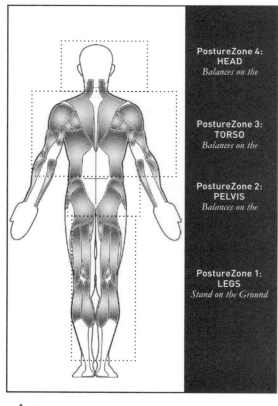

PostureZone 4:
HEAD
Balances on the

PostureZone 3:
TORSO
Balances on the

PostureZone 2:
PELVIS
Balances on the

PostureZone 1:
LEGS
Stand on the Ground

▲ **Figure 6-8** The 4 Posture Zones

Trick Motions

Trick motions are when you cheat and use one motion at the expense of another. These adaptations to normal movement may begin when you favored a knee because of an injury, from learning poor form when golfing, or even from slumping poor posture as a child. Unconscious posture and motion control occurs at each individual joint, as well as from the brain's control of posture. However, our body thinks in terms of whole motions, not individual muscles. So, when you favor one joint motion at the expense of another, you are moving other muscles and joints adaptively, and less effectively.

> **A change in one link of the chain forces different alignment of other links.**

Like the folds on a piece of paper, your unique BodyType, your injuries, and LifeHabits literally become part of how your body moves. If you sleep on your stomach with your head turned to the right, when standing you will find you head does not turn as easily to the left. When you prop a phone under your neck while talking, your neck twists more easily to that side. If you sit on the wallet you keep in your right hip pocket or always carry a purse on your right shoulder, it doesn't feel right when you put it on your left side. Just like a piece of cardboard, tissues hold their crease.

Many people with back problems say they have poor posture. They are usually right. Studies show people with chronic low back pain actually move with specifically different patterns of motion, even when they are not in acute pain[xxxiv], according to high-tech scientific research as well as the clinical observations of many posture professionals.

If a learned motion is called muscle memory, then a forgotten motion should be called muscle amnesia. Just as we use positive muscle memory to perform a task unconsciously, negative muscle memory keeps us doing things the same wrong way. We are completely unaware that there is another way to move, which is why every good personal trainer, exercise instructor, physical therapist, and chiropractor stresses proper form when teaching exercises.

"Practice doesn't make perfect, practice makes permanent."

Over time, when the motion of individual joints is limited, motion changes affect the alignment and the fit of the joint surfaces, eventually causing injury, pain, and arthritic breakdown. Much of the benefit from a chiropractic adjustment comes from the manipulation of a misaligned joint to reduce this mechanical stress and restore full range motion.

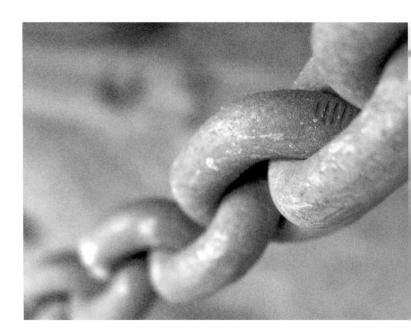

▲ **Figure 6-9** Chain of Motion

In a chain (including the kinetic chain of body motion) the tightest link will restrict overall motion. Loose links move before tight links. So, if you are a chiropractor adjusting a spine or a yoga teacher showing StrongPosture™ exercises, to focus a stretch on a tight area you must first take out all the tension from the adjacent, more freely moveable areas. This is why performing StrongPosture™ exercises and stretches feels "weird" at first. You are literally moving your body in a different way, like a folded piece of cardboard being bent right next to a crease.

To stretch the tight link in a chain of motion, you must stretch it last.

Once you learn to consciously train new paths of motion and feel the inner strength of stable posture, you begin to unconsciously integrate new motion patterns into your daily life. The result: stronger posture with less strain on muscles and joints.

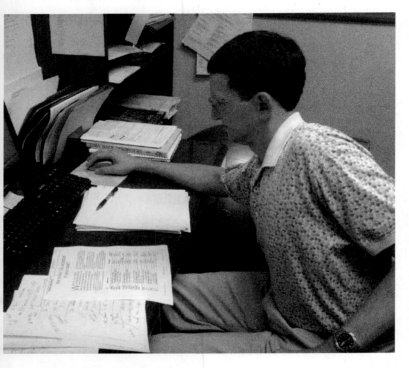

▲ **Figure 6-10** The body folds in predictable patterns when kept in a stressed position

StrongPosture™ for Winning Performance

Performance depends on form, which depends on Strong-Posture™ . Every sports trainer and coach teaches about form. Good form is StrongPosture™ in motion, which is why StrongPosture™ is integral to performance.

Ideal form is using the body to optimize the effectiveness without overstressing and straining any muscle or joint in the kinetic chain. When you are in motion you shift in and out of balance so you must maintain equilibrium, so good form requires strong core muscles to fight gravity's pull.

Balance and stability are two sides of the same coin. If you are running and don't get your foot in front of you quickly enough, you fall down. If you are golfing and do not shift your weight correctly, you will instinctively move your foot to "keep your balance." A golf swing is a whole pattern, which is why golfers know lifting your head will ruin a shot. Baseball player or cyclist, worker or parent lifting a child out of a car seat: all balance their bodies as a whole for the activity in which they are engaged.

A frequent frustration for athletes is when they practice but don't get better. The reason is they think are doing one thing, but in reality are doing something quite different. In tennis, golf, and all other sports, the ball always agrees with reality.

When you think about it, posture is not just about how you stand; it is also about how your body moves and balances in everything you do.

In every sport, balance is a tremendous factor in winning. Great athletes have great balance and control of their bodies' motion. Michael Jordan made it look easy when he shot a basketball because he balanced perfectly and controlled his body motion as he jumped to guide the ball in the basket, and then returned gracefully to the ground.

Olympic figure skaters balance on a knife's edge, football players run and dodge, and golfers use their bodies to get the head of a golf club moving with a perfect trajectory to precisely impact a ball so it travels over 300 yards.

While world-class athletes have precision control of their bodies, research shows that StrongPosture™ and balance improves performance and efficiency for just about any physical activity. StrongPosture™ exercise is not just for helping elite athletes perform better: walker or runner, yoga practitioner or tennis player, exercising with Strong-Posture™ adds to the health benefits of your exercise.

For more on patterns see www.bodyzone.com/Patterns

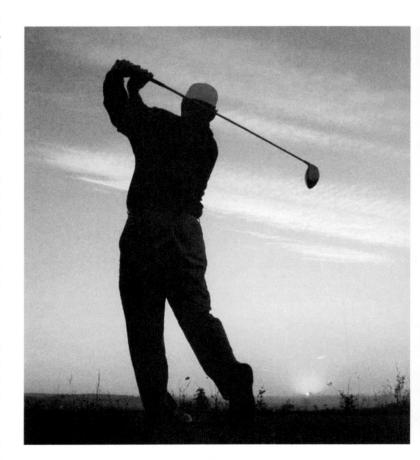

 Figure 6-11 Good form!

120|

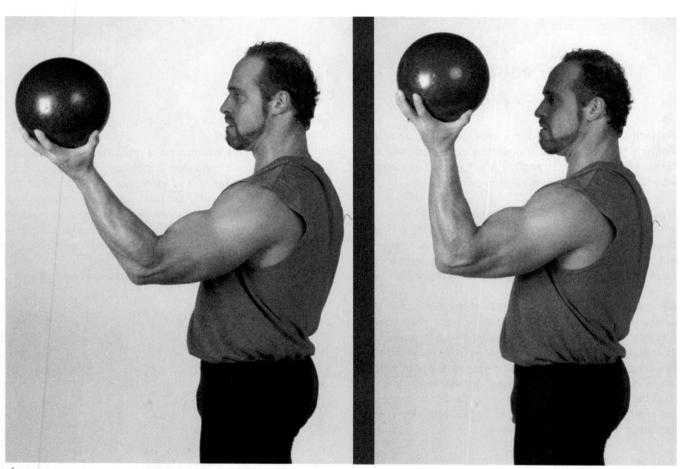

▲ **Figure 6-12** It's harder to hold up a bowling ball (or a head) when it's not well balanced.

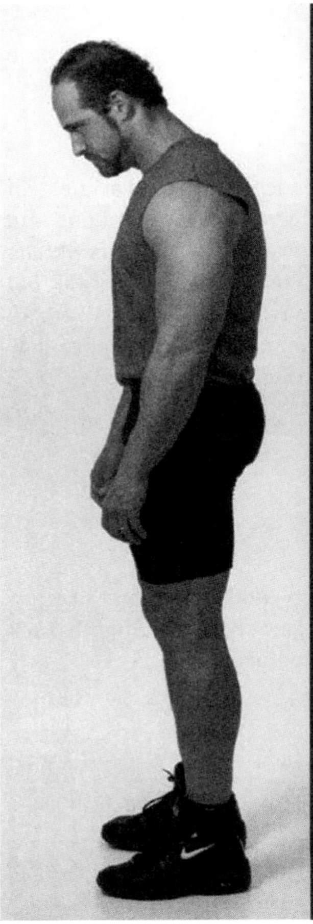

Figure 6-13 Poorly balanced head posture creates neck strain

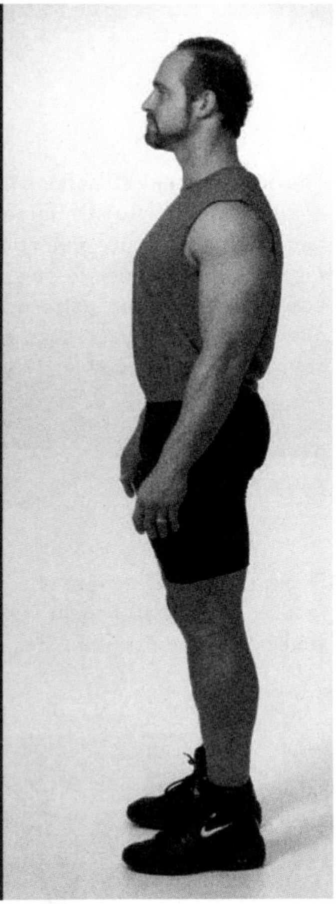

Figure 6-14 StrongPosture™: Pelvis tucked, head back

StrongPosture™ Alignment:
Neck Retractions

Keeping a Level Head on Your Shoulders

After learning breath and pelvic control, the next StrongPosture™ exercise is to learn to control the head. Often, when you retrain one part of the body's motion, something else shifts to compensate. We saw how it becomes harder to balance a weight when it moves out of alignment when we balanced the golf club. Imagine a fifteen-pound bowling ball (about the weight of a human head) balanced on a seven-inch rod (such as the neck). If the ball is shifted forward, it takes dramatically more energy to keep the ball up.

Research studies show that for every inch forward of center the head is balanced, the effective weight of the head being carried by the neck and shoulder muscles doubles!

It's not surprising that people with forward head posture complain their neck muscles are tired!

122|

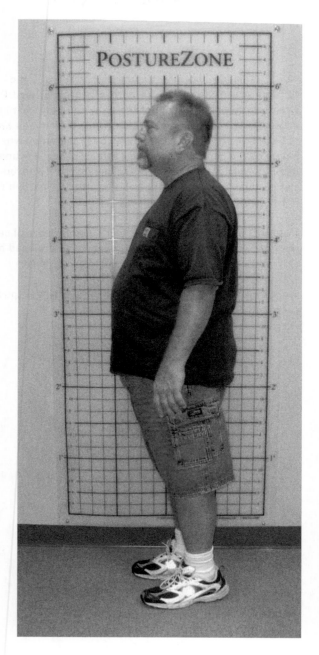

The goal of neck retractions is to increase the awareness of head position while strengthening your control of head and neck motion. Posture distortions are neurological as well as mechanical. In order to strengthen balance and break old posture and motion patterns, you must become aware of how you balance your head on your torso and consciously connect head motion to pelvis motion.

THE EXERCISE
AWARE POSTION

Begin in a WallTilt; feet shoulder-width apart and about a foot from the wall as you lean against a wall. Slightly tuck your pelvis and maintain StrongPosture™.

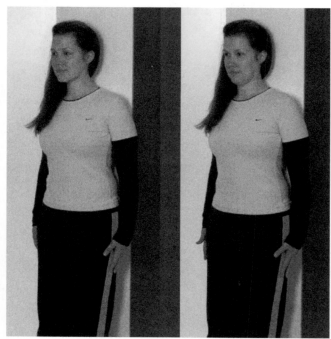

Figure 6-15 Weak posture: pelvis forward, head forward

Figure 6-16 Neck Retraction A,B

Now, let your shoulders drop, and pull the tips of your shoulder blades in toward your spine. Look straight ahead and keep your head and chin level.

CONSCIOUS MOTION

Slowly press your head straight back toward the wall, and then let it glide easily forward. Maintain a pelvic tilt, and use 5 slow breaths to control your motion.

1) Breathe out and press your head toward the wall
  Keep your chin level and look straight ahead
  Breathe in and let your head gently glide slightly forward
  Keep your head level

2) Breathe out and try to touch your head to the wall
  Move as though your head is on railroad tracks, keeping it level
  Breathe in and let your head gently glide forward
  Breathe slowly, letting your breath control your motion

3) Breathe out and pull your head backward
  Keep your pelvis tucked under as you make your neck and spine long
  Breathe in slowly
  Look at a point straight ahead of you as your head goes forward

4) Breathe out and press your head firmly toward the wall
  Keep your shoulders down and arms at your side as you lengthen your spine
  Breathe in
  Move as slowly as you can and touch each degree of motion

5) Breathe out and feel your head rising toward the ceiling
  Tuck your pelvis as your neck stretches and lengthens your spine
  Breathe in, gently glide forward

≫TRY THIS: *Feeling where you look*

When you look at something, even before you turn your head, the deep neck muscles contract, which is why eye position is important to effectively re-train the patterns that control body movement. Poker players watch their opponents' eyes and body for unconscious "tells" because the body and mind work together.

Controlling where you look is important when doing StrongPosture™ exercises because these muscles work with the deep, core muscles of the body to stabilize and balance the body. These deep neck muscles are literally wired directly to the eyes, so when people learn to stabilize their neck, many continue to shift stress by looking up instead of straight ahead.

When doing neck retractions (or pelvic tilts), it is important to look straight ahead and focus on a fixed point to keep your head level.

To feel the contraction of these deep neck muscles:
  Put 2 fingers at the top of the neck, just under the ridge of the skull.
  Without moving your head, slow look as far to the left as you can.
      You will feel the motion of the neck muscles preparing to turn your head even though only your eyes have moved.
  Try looking to the right, left, up and down, and feel which neck muscles work.
So if you spend your day looking down at a computer screen, you're working the neck muscles that cause Forward Head Posture and other posture problems.

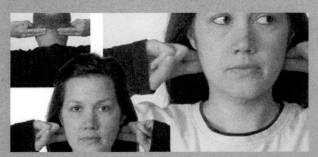

▲ **Figure 6-17** The deep neck muscles work to stabilize the neck as you move your eyes

¹²⁴ *PEELBACKS:*

A. The purpose of neck retractions is to strengthen the body's perception of the head being balanced over the shoulders, so it is important to press the head toward the wall, but only gently. Explore the forward motion of the head. It is far more important to keep the head level than to touch the wall.

B. Try doing Necks Retractions with a mirror. Look straight ahead. Put a finger on your chin to consciously keep your head level. Press your head straight back, visualizing the motion of your head to be a train moving on railroad tracks. Don't look up. Then, keep your face level as you glide your neck forward with your breath.

C. Do neck retractions slowly for five slow breaths, twice a day, moving consciously while holding your pelvis firmly in a tuck.

If you have a clinical symptom such as neck pain, shoulder problems, or headaches, doing a neck retraction may be difficult or painful. If so, only move within the pain-free range of motion. In many posture distortions, before a muscle can be strengthened with focused exercises, the shortened tight ligaments, adhesions, and muscles need to be gently lengthened. If pain persists, see a professional.

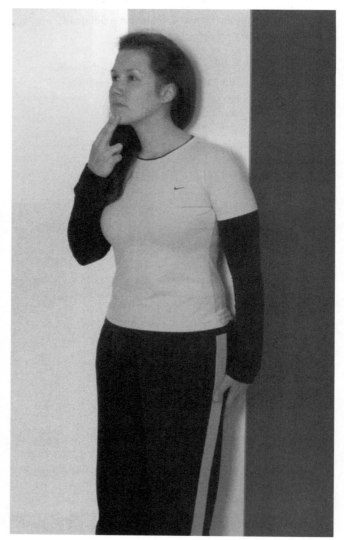

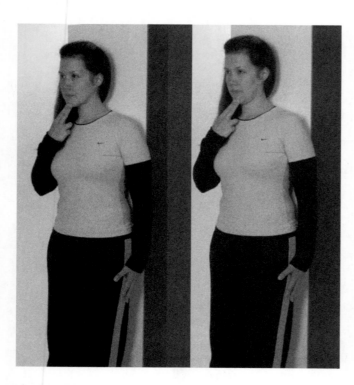

▲ **Figure 6-18** Correct cervical retractions

▲ **Figure 6-19** Incorrect cervical retractions

Towel Roll assisted neck retraction.

If you have a severe Forward Head Posture and cannot come close to touching the wall without looking up, place a rolled-up towel behind your head. Keep it in place by pressing it against the wall as you tuck your chin to level your head. Repeat 5 times.

For an additional challenge, instead of a towel try using a tennis ball.

PROGRESSIONS:
Tip of your tongue

Think about your tongue: where is it in your mouth right now? You may not realize it, but tongue position and motion can be restricted by posture problems.

TIP: Press the tip of your tongue to the roof of your mouth as you press your neck into retraction and see if you can't stretch your neck a bit farther back.

Lateral neck stretch

Do a neck retraction. While the neck is pulled back, and keeping the face forward, slowly stretch the neck to the side. DO NOT turn your head toward the floor. When done correctly you should feel a deep neck stretch (especially in commonly tight muscles called levator scapula).

Clinical Tip for Sleepy Arms

If you ever have your hand or arm fall asleep, next time this happens an easy fix is to simply change your posture.

Stand up (thereby changing the support for the neck) and bend your neck left and right to reduce pressure on the nerves in the neck from bones and muscles. Do this back and forth ten times, keeping your face forward while breathing and moving slowly. It may not be as good as a chiropractic adjustment or massage, but I've seen this trick help many people with neck problems and "pins and needles" (sleepy limbs).

126|

StrongPosture™ Alignment:
Variations: LockBacks
and SeeSaw

If you have a forward head posture, you likely noticed a strong tendency to look toward the ceiling when doing pelvic tucks. This postural chain pulling your head up and extending your neck is from shortening and stretching opposing muscles and ligaments, especially in the spine.

Lengthening the spine is a common goal of yoga, Pilates, or any posture strengthening exercise. The spine is the centerline chain of our body. When moving a chain, the tightest link will move last. To move that tight link, you need to either support the loose links or lock them by moving them to the end of their range of motion. When stretching a chain, the last thing stretched is going to stretch the most.

When tucking the pelvis, you are pulling down on the bottom end of the spinal chain. When you do a neck retraction you are pulling on the now stiffest link in the chain so you feel more stretch there. On the other hand, if you do a neck retraction first and stretch the top of the chain, and you will find more tension when then doing a pelvic tilt to stretch the other end of the chain.

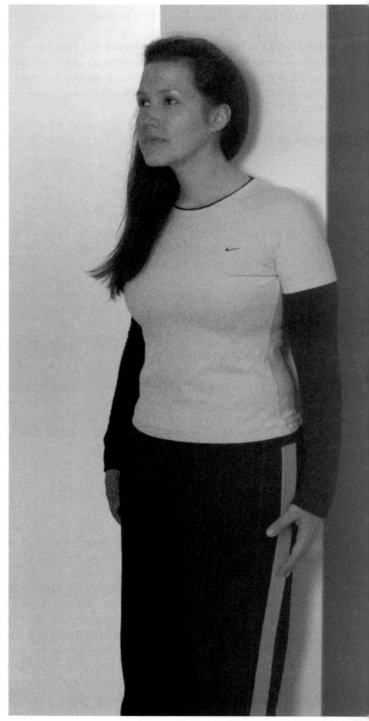

▲ **Figure 6-20** Incorrect WallTilt tuck with neck extension

»TRY THIS: *This Way or That Way Stretch*

The This Way or That Way demo will help you get a feel for how posture changes affect what area is stressed when you do a stretch.

Stand straight

Keeping your knees locked and straight, bend down to touch your left toe.

Where do you feel the stretch?

After straightening, now bend your left knee 30°, and bend forward (palm the floor or touch your knee... just get as low as you can)

Then, keeping your pelvis tucked as far as you can, straighten your knees.

Now where do you feel the stretch?

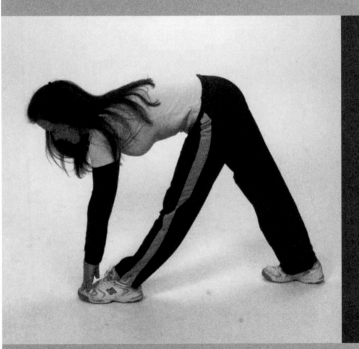

▲ **Figure 6-21a** Straight leg toe touch

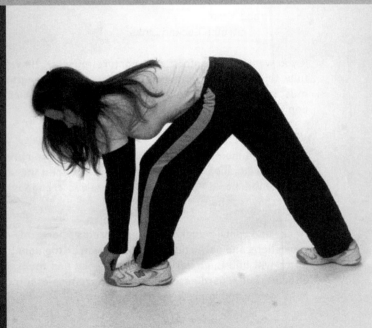

▲ **Figure 6-21b** Bent leg toe touch

128|

Abnormal patterns of joint movement create patterns of muscle and joint tightness that "lock" a person into their postures and motion patterns. One way doctors of chiropractic can so effectively help change motion patterns is by adjusting the spine to unlock key spinal links and restore motion to relieve tension on the spinal chain.

Posture changes cause tension on the spinal chain. The seesawing of your neck looking up when you tuck your pelvis, or your low back arching when you tuck your neck is like a child's playground teeter totter: both sides can't be up at the same time. Like two children playing, when you push down on one side of a seesaw, the other side comes up.

Many exercises don't effectively target the weak link of a chain because, when you move, you instinctively UNstress the weakest link in a kinetic chain to use your strong muscles. To strengthen a weak link you have to use your body in a way to STRESS that link, which can often be exactly opposite of how you instinctively move.

In other words, to effectively stretch a tight link in the postural chain:
> First,
>> Lock Stretched Links,
> and Then
>> Stretch Locked Links

If you want to strengthen core posture muscles, they must fully lengthen and then contract. You can't strengthen a muscle fiber that works in an angle of motion in which you don't move.

> **Clinical Note: If you are thinking, "AH-HA- what about isometric vs isokinetic exercise?", you are not a casual reader and the answer is beyond the scope of this book. For more info, see www.strongposture. com/isokinetic**

Neck and pelvic lockbacks are progressions of neck retractions and pelvic tilts to focus stretch on the tight links. Some will find them very easy, some may find them more difficult, but regardless, increased awareness of a motion helps refine and improve form.

■ A: Neck LockBack (Strong Neck)

GOAL: Maintain neck retraction while doing a focused pelvic tilt to become aware of and strengthen control of the motion between the pelvis, head, and the torso.

AWARE POSTION:
Focused Pelvic Tilt position, against the wall, with your back straight, feet shoulder-width apart, about a foot from the wall.
Pull the tips of your shoulder blades together, gently squeezing them toward your spine.

Conscious Motion:
Pull your neck back into a neck retraction.
Then, as you firmly lock your neck back, flatten your low back in a strong pelvic tuck.
Continue holding your neck back, and then slowly arch your low back in a pelvic arch.

> Breathe IN as the pelvis rolls forward and pull the neck into a strong retraction, keeping the chin level.
> Breathe OUT as the pelvis rolls back, keeping the head locked back.

Breath and motion should be smooth and synchronized.
Repeat, and do 5 Pelvic Tilts and Arches as you keep your neck pressed firmly into the wall.

> Note: Where do you feel the stretch?

Tip: Press your big toe into the floor and strengthen your pelvic tuck as you breathe out and press your neck back.

■ B: Pelvic LockBack (Strong Pelvis)

Goal: Hold a strong, full pelvic tuck firmly as you do neck retractions.
Keeping a pelvic tuck

> Breathe in and gently let your neck glide forward
> Breathe out and press your neck back.

As you breathe out and tuck, press your big toe into the floor and roll your thighs in to strengthen your pelvic lock.
Note: Where do you feel the stretch?

■ C: SEESaw Stretch:
Stretch Everything Evenly

I129

Alternate between locking your pelvis back as you do a neck retraction, and locking your neck in retraction as you do a pelvic tuck. Note: Where do you feel the stretch?

With lock and stretch exercises, the goal is FIRST lock A, THEN stretch B.

Move slowly and smoothly, allowing your breath to pace your motion. If your motion is not smooth, if you are "skipping" parts of the arc of motion, try to move as slowly as possible through all of that arc of motion.

Alternating between pushing one side of the "seesaw" down, and then the other, is a lock- and stretch-focused motion exercise to help you Stretch Everything Evenly.

Proper form allows you to strengthen normal movement patterns.

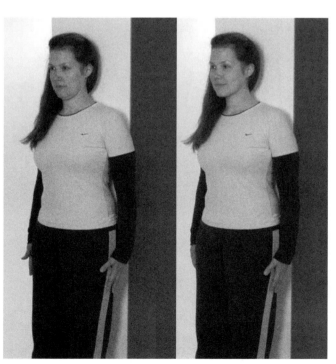

▲ **Figure 6-22** SeeSaw

130|

Abs and StrongPosture™

Abdominal weakness is a major factor in low back pain. Weak core and lower abdominal muscles ("pouchy" belly) strain the back and create myriad postural problems. Unfortunately, even though people talk about strong abs many exercise routines work the hip flexors (large muscles which bend the hip) far more than the abs. In addition, research shows that many people with "six-pack" abs may frequently suffer back pain because they have trained their body to work only one part of the abs and so have poor control of pelvic motion.

In fact, low back pain correlates with a loss of use of the deepest part of the abdominals, the transverse abs (TrA), as compared to the rest of the abs[xxxv]. Effective low back exercises must focus on these often neglected and weak muscles (transverse abdominus, oblique and/or external abdominal muscles)[xxxvi].

»TRY THIS: *Belly In or Out*

Is your ab exercise working your abs or your hip flexors (psoas)?
To find out, do a sit-up (or abdominal crunch).
Look at your belly as you come up.

> If your belly stays flat or goes slightly in, you are using your abs—a great thing.
> If your belly pushes out, sorry, but you are working your hip flexors.

Think about it: When muscles contract they get shorter. If you use your abs to lift the torso, the belly goes flat or pulls in. If you sit a lot your hip flexors are probably tight, and so your patterns of motion use them and avoid the weak abs.

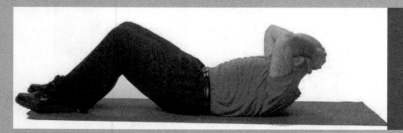

Figure 6-23a Belly-in works abs   ▲   **Figure 6-23b** Belly-out uses hip flexors to avoid working abs

StrongPosture™ Motion: AbFocus - Strengthening core abdominal control of pelvic motion

The ball-based AbFocus requires you to stabilize and balance to contract the abs through a fuller range of motion. A fuller range of motion means more muscle fibers are working than traditional situps or crunches where you start flexing from flat on the floor.

Also, AbFocus helps you find and work unused fibers by consciously moving in a controlled, coupled sequence.

Controlled AbFocus exercises target the abs to effectively strengthen posture and balance adaptive patterns of motion. Beginning an AbFocus (or any exercise) with a strong pelvis (or a slight pelvic tilt) changes how all the other muscles in the body stabilize. When you use a strong pelvis you hold the torso stable, then move the hips up by pulling the stomach in, and then flex the neck and the torso. With traditional ab exercises, the hips are down making it easier to use your hip flexors to pull the torso up.

GOAL
Fully contract and lengthen abdominals by starting with the torso extended and abs lengthened in a BallStretch, then progressively and fully contracting the abs into a crunch by pulling the abdominals in with control, and then slowly lengthening them as you go down.

AWARE POSITION:
From BackStretch, roll forward into a comfortable squat. Keep your buttocks on the ball and bend your knees until your torso is at a comfortable 45° or so angle.
The more vertical you are on the ball, the easier an AbFocus is to do. The farther back on the ball you stretch, the more you work the abs along their full length as you fully extend the torso and then contract the abs.
Place your left hand on top of your left shoulder, and your right hand on your right shoulder.
Keep your elbows shoulder width apart.

CONTROLLED MOTION:
The goal of AbFocus is sequential and smooth motion using deep core muscle control.

Each motion of AbFocus should be independent but smoothly connected. Think of a zipper moving one link at a time as you ZipUP and ZipDown with progressive contraction to find unused muscle fibers and patterns.

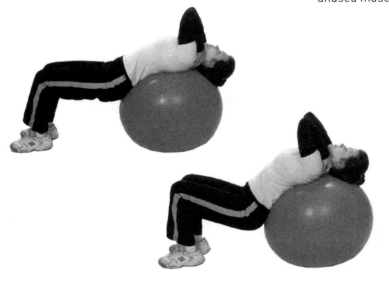
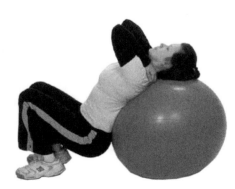

▲ **Figure 6-24** AbFocus Aware Position

▲ **Figure 5-xx AbFocus Aware Position**

132| *AbFocus ZipUP, with slow, controlled motion*

First: Tuck the pelvis
>   Pull the belly in (hollowing) to lift the hips.
>   >   Don't roll the ball.
>   >   Don't move your knees to "bridge"- this uses your quads instead of your abs.

then: Bring the chin to the chest.
then: Bring your nose toward your belly button.
then: Squeeze the stomach into an AbFocus Crunch.
>   Keep your belly button pulled into your spine as you
pull the lower ribs to the top of the hips.

ZipDOWN, with slow, controlled motion

Keeping your belly in and pelvis tucked
First: Drop your shoulders to the ball as you keep your chin to your chest.
then: Let the head touch the ball, keeping the belly in and hips up.
then: Smoothly drop the pelvis.
then: Smoothly let the belly fully relax.
>   IMPORTANT: To target unused, deep muscle fibers completely drop the pelvis and fully relax the tuck so the abs can fully lengthen (before they have to shorten again as you ZipUP).

>   People with weak TrA and lower abs will often unconsciously hold the pelvis up to avoid having to contract them again.

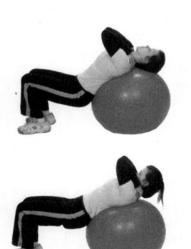
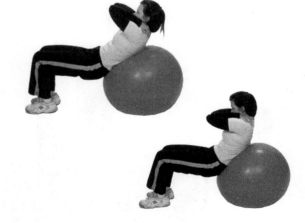
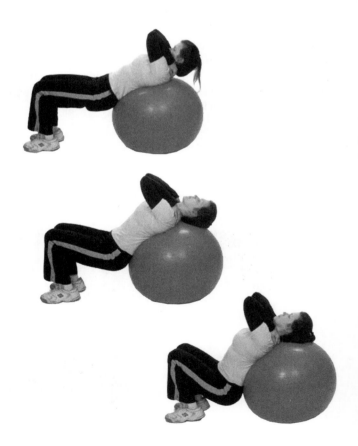

▲ **Figure 6-25** AbFocus ZipUP

▲ **Figure 6-26** AbFocus ZipDOWN

BREATHING

Breathe from the lower abs.
Press the lower abs to the spine using the ZipUp motion.
Breathe OUT as you slowly curl UP into a crunch. Breathe IN as you slowly curl DOWN in a BackStretch over the ball.

Repetitions

Ab strength varies tremendously. Start with 5 repetitions and increase as your stamina allows with strong form. Do only as many as you can do with full control.

The Core, the Pelvic Floor, and Kegels

Incorporate pelvic floor exercise into AbFocus by beginning the ZipUp with tightening the rectal and urinary control muscles (think of stopping the stream when you are urinating). This is a deep contraction, not to be confused with tightening the buttocks, and should begin before the pelvis is lifted and then stay contracted until after the pelvis is dropped.

ZipUP from the bottom and hollow belly as you breathe out and:

> Kegel
> Pelvic lift
> Chin to chest
> Shoulder lift
> Squeeze abs (belly button to spine) and Kegel muscles

Then breathe in and ZipDown using the abs for controlled motion, from the top and with controlled relaxation (no sudden drops)

> Drop shoulders
> Head to ball
> Pelvic Drop
> Relax Abs
> Relax Kegel

Think of it as an internal zipper that begins deep in your pelvis and zips up and in to hold your lower abdominal contents in place, just like zipping up a pair of trousers with a very long, very low zipper.

PEELBACKS:

Use your forearms to support your head.
Roll down on the ball so your body approaches a 90°
angle to the floor.

▼ **Figure 6-27** Low AbFocus

PROGRESSIONS:

Roll up on the ball so your body approaches level with the
floor.

Also, see BallHug progression for AbCrunch and other ab
exercises in Chapter 8.

▼ **Figure 6-28** High AbFocus

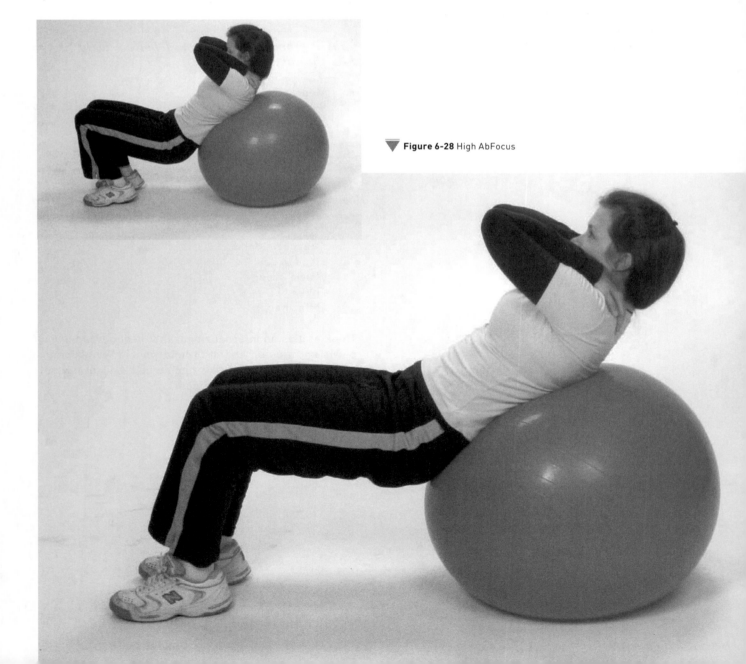

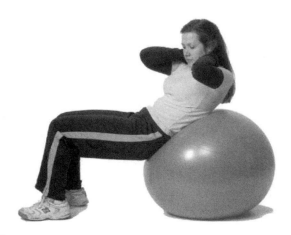

LifeHabits

While StrongPosture™ exercises are uniquely valuable, you need to do more to stay healthy. Along with balance and motion exercises, cardiovascular, strength, and flexibility training are also essential for good health.

There are lots of paths to good health, but one of the easiest and most accessible exercises is as old as man: walking. Walking is an ideal exercise for the human frame. The incidence of injury is minimal, and the benefits are significant.

Tip: Use StrongPosture™ next time you take a walk.
     Focus on posture by holding a slight pelvic tuck for
     5 Breaths

▲ **Figure 6-29** Crossed AbFocus

▼ **Figure 6-30** Wide Legged AbFocus

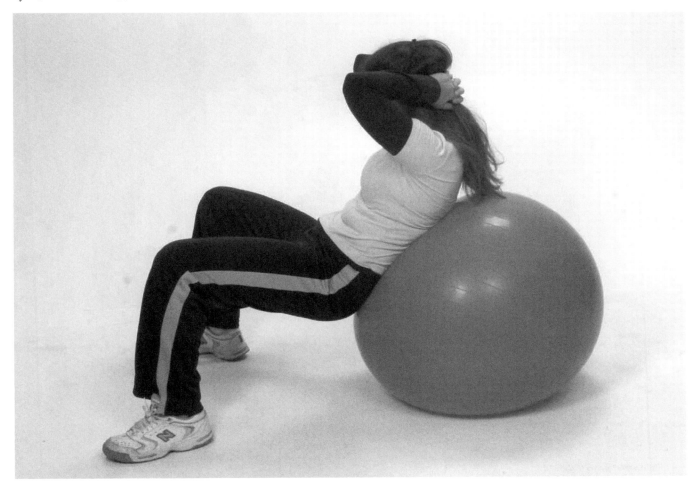

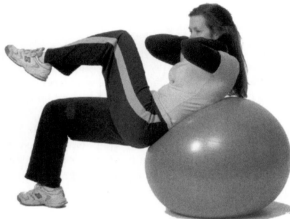

Figure 6-31 AbFocus Cross with leg lift

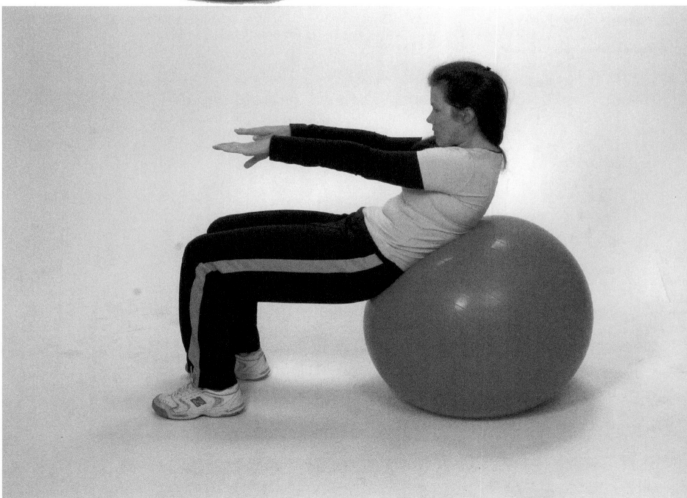

Figure 6-32 Arms to Ceiling

StrongPosture™
7 Week Program-

B

A

M

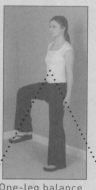

One-leg balance
(**The Stork**)-p.19

Strong Balance

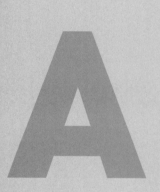

WallTilt -p66

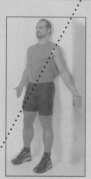

Neck Retractions
-p.122

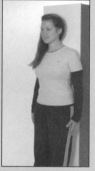

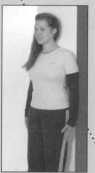

SeeSaw -p.129

Strong Alignment

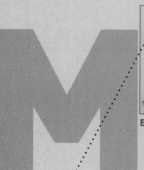

BallTilt Arch -p.75

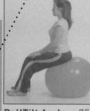

BallTilt Tuck -p.75

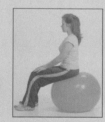

BallStretch -p.101

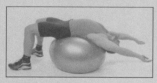

AbFocus -p.132

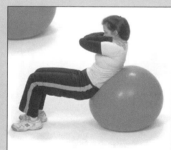

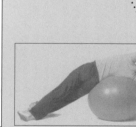

SideStretch -p.103

Strong Motion

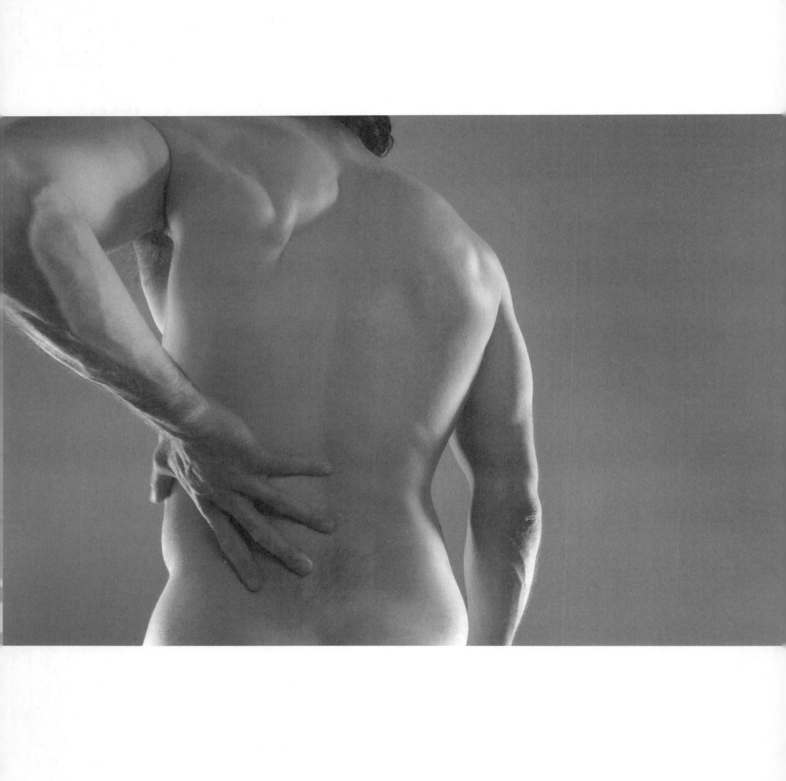

7 Compensation
The 4th Posture Principle

The Body Learns to Move in the Patterns You Teach It...AND Pain Teaches the Body to Move Differently

In the race of life, the person running with one shoe off and one shoe on is a lot less likely to win. S.Weiniger

Did you know there are computer keyboards on which you can type faster, with less risk of motion problems such as carpal tunnel syndrome? It's true, but there is no market for these alternative keyboards because we all learned to type on a standard QWERTY keyboard, with keys placed to prevent old-fashioned typewriter arms from jamming if we typed too fast.

140| Our keyboards (and our bodies) were not designed with computers in mind, but even though it may not be best, we all work on a keyboard designed for a typewriter because our bodies learned to move in the patterns in which we trained them to move.

We have seen how motion, a basic property of all living things, is the first Posture Principle. Balance is the second, and is of especially great significance to humans because we balance on two feet instead of the four that nature provides most other creatures.

Patterns, the third principle, governs the motion of all creatures, and 21st century human bodies suffer the unique stress of living in relatively narrow ranges of motion. Technology allows us to enhance our ability and productivity but focuses us on limited sets of motions. The human frame is designed to move in an incredibly complex dance where even the simplest motions are composed of the interactions of hundreds of muscles working together in an infinite variety of possible combinations. However, we live most of our lives in a small fraction of the potential motions our muscles and joints can move in.

The factory worker in an assembly line, the cook flipping burgers, the construction worker hammering, or the computer worker staring at a screen and hitting the same keys all day (albeit in a different order) are all deepening the grooves of their patterns of motion. And of course, our sitting society keeps our torso and head bent forward like an old person. After we sit driving and sit at work, we go home to relax and sit motionless in front of a TV.

Muscles and joints work specifically at different angles and in different combinations, and become trained (learn) to move in whatever patterns you move in. When you shrug your shoulder when typing the angle of the shoulder to the torso is slightly changed, forcing the elbow to compensate and the wrist to shift to keep your fingers on the keys. This changes the angles at which muscles are working, and fires different sets of muscle fibers. The dance of our body's motion is called a kinetic chain for good reason. Our motion is the result of multiple muscles contracting to move, assist, and stabilize multiple bones at multiple joints.

Posture, or how you balance your body, is such a chain. From the ankles to the knees, from the pelvis to the chest, and from the shoulders to the head, every link in the chain moves

in a pattern dependent upon, and in relation to, whatever it's connected to. If your habit is to keep the shoulders forward of your hips, the front of the ribcage is going to pull you forward and down. When you try to "sit up straight," you must use your back muscles in a mechanically inefficient and unsustainable way.

> And within the postural chain of motion, at the end of it all, the net sum of weights and forces MUST balance...or we fall down.
>
> And maintaining balance takes individual muscle fibers either being fully contracted, or not, with nerves telling each fiber to contract, or not.

This brings us to the fact that many people believe they are standing straight and erect with good posture even though a camera shows they are not. When you took your posture picture (I am assuming you have already done so...if not, try it as soon as you can), you may have observed you were not standing as straight as you thought you were. For most people, when it comes to posture (and many other things in life), there is a difference between perceptions and reality.

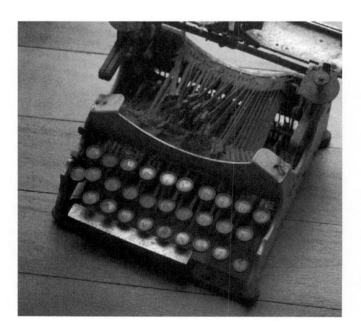

▲ **Figure 7-1** Typewriter with jammed keys

The Cycles of Life

For every action there is an equal and opposite reaction. Newton's 3rd Law of Motion

Everything is caused by actions and reactions. Actions have reactions, which in turn become causes of other actions. Living systems occur when a cycle is formed from a chain of actions and reactions.

From tides to hemlines, from stock markets to weather cycles, everything rises and falls in inexorable cycles. The moon goes around the earth, and the earth 'round the sun in an ongoing cycle. There are economic and business cycles, as well as cycles when we look at health or human behaviors. When we look at the cycles of health, there are behavioral, psychological, and biological factors that all contribute to various cycles, both vicious and virtuous.

Cycles are everywhere in nature and in living systems. We learned in high school that life on our planet depends on the cycle of photosynthesis. Every animal cell is powered by the energy of the Krebs Cycle. And even though he didn't invent it, Al Gore summarized well the complex interactions of living eco-systems on Earth as being cyclic. Plants take in carbon from carbon dioxide and create sugars, which are then consumed by animals, which feed the plants by exhaling carbon dioxide.

From the large to the small, in nature things work in cycles. An American naturalist, William Beebe, was exploring the jungles of Guyana when he came upon a circle of army ants, 1,200 feet around. It took each ant two and a half hours to make one revolution! Each ant was simply following the ant in front, as they all went 'round and 'round, until most of the ants died.

Ants are not necessarily aware, and insofar as our health, posture, and body motion are concerned, most of the time neither are we.

Is it lack of exercise and motion that causes back pain, or is it that people with back problems don't move and exercise? Cycles may have no clear beginning, or even direction. Which comes first, the chicken or the egg? This is the problem with defining an easy solution for many problems, including posture problems or back pain.

142|

Health and Posture Cycles

> *The musculo-skeletal system comprises roughly 60 percent of the structure of the human body, and it expends most of the energy of the body.* Leon Chaitow

People who are physically active stay fit. People who are fit, by and large, feel good. And people who feel good are able to stay physically active. The most important thing you do, from your body's point of view, is to keep moving. After all, the ability to get from here to there, or locomotion, is the reason for existence of the body's largest system, and consumes the most energy of any system in the body.

It may seem obvious, but one cycle of health is:

On the other hand, people who are inactive generally do not exercise. Over time, their bodies weaken. When they try to do physical activity, they tire easily, reinforcing the habit of inactivity. Since posture is such an important indicator of good health, it is not surprising that there are cycles that affect posture. We are born loose and we die stiff. As we age, worsening posture and motion can make us look, feel, and act old, even while we are still young. The accumulation of chronic inactivity plus the micro-traumas of living within restricted patterns of motion cause changes that, while microscopic and initially imperceptible, add up to cumulative changes in tissue elasticity, flexibility, and tensile strength. Combine this with imperfectly healed injuries, and slowly you begin to say, "I'm not as young as I once was," or "I just can't do what I used to do."

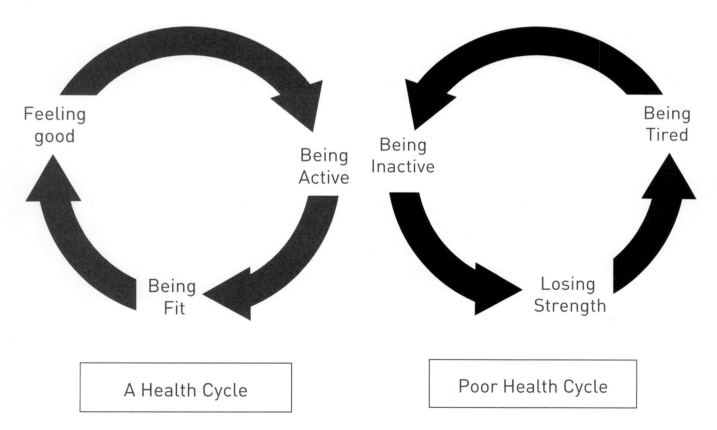

Feeling good → Being Active → Being Fit → Feeling good

A Health Cycle

Being Inactive → Being Tired → Losing Strength → Being Inactive

Poor Health Cycle

▲ **Figure 7-2** Health Cycle

▲ **Figure 7-3** Poor Health Cycle

Loss of motion is a loss of vitality as well as a loss of function. But, before you label yourself with the self-fulfilling prophecy of "I am just old," stop and think about this: How many times have you lived with mild, "normal" pain? If you can fill in the blank for "I have a weak _____," whether your problem area (or limiting factor) is in the back, neck, shoulder, or knee, your body's motion patterns have adapted for that weakness. These adaptations result in further injury when you push against newly restrictive limits of joint motion and weakened strength.

It's obvious when you stop and think about it that if a muscle is moving differently, the motion of the associated joint will also be different. Similarly, if a joint is moving differently, the associated muscle(s) are functioning differently. And when these two hands clasp together, we have a cycle:

Poor posture means the body must move differently. And different motions of the body will have an effect on posture. In other words,

The body learns to move in ways you teach it

In Patterns, the 3rd Posture Principle, we saw how trick motions are blind spots of motion, a gap between perception and reality, which is one of the reasons people are oblivious to posture asymmetries and problems. The biomechanical stress of spending half your life folded in a sitting position is also compounded by any injury you suffered as your body learned to move in ways to avoid that pain. The problem is, when the pain goes away, people often continue moving in a way to avoid the pain, even after it is gone. Muscle imbalance, joint stress, and pain can result from trying to avoid pain, and then the asymmetric motion can stress joints and cause pain with no new injury.

In my chiropractic practice I have seen many patients who present with excruciating low back pain from something as inconsequential as bending over to pick up a nickel. These "back attack" patients are frequently experiencing the results of living with ignored or low-grade pain. And after the attack subsides, their motion is just a bit more adaptive, taking them another step on a vicious cycle of adaptive motion. After literally decades of periodic episodes in a long-term spiral, many of these people eventually tell me they are "old" now. Like an army ant walking in a big circle,

144| they rationalize their age as the reason they just can't do what they used to. The fact is, a large part of slowly creating their "old" body was the sum of each day's activities, or their habits, and never mind that someone else ten years older feels and acts twenty years younger. The loss of function happens too slowly to see, like the hour hand on a watch or the setting sun. By the time many people stop and think about their vitality, all they can do is wonder, "Where did it go?"

For many, many people, our 21st century sedentary sitting lifestyle is a root cause of feeling and acting old far earlier than nature intended. Sitting uses muscles in a way that creates biomechanical stress in order to maintain balance as the body uses some muscles too much and others too little. A vicious cycle of unbalanced motion, adaptation, and breakdown results, which in turn causes more unbalanced motion and muscle fatigue. Years of inactivity cause progressive adaptive changes that result in weakening the body's strength and balance. Thus begins the Pain Cycle, a vicious spiral of poor posture and unbalanced motion causing chronic pain and recurring injury.

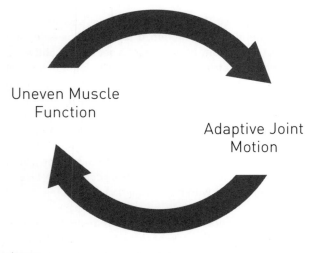

▲ **Figure 7-4** Muscles and adaptive motion

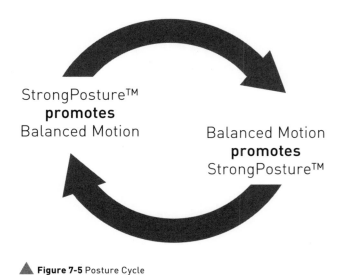

▲ **Figure 7-5** Posture Cycle

The Pain Cycle

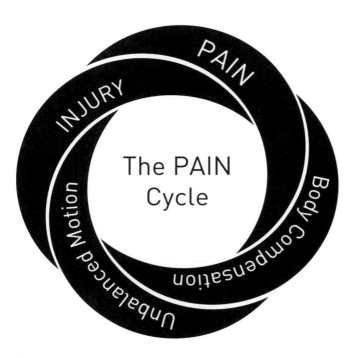

▲ **Figure 7-6** Pain Cycle

The Pain Cycle is when injury causes pain.

    Then the pain causes the body to compensate.

        Then, the body's compensation results in unbalanced motion, which sets the stage for injury and posture to worsen.

            The adaptation of unbalanced motion and poor posture stresses joints and muscles, causing premature wear and predisposing the joint to injury.

These Pain Cycle concepts are basic explanations of ideas taught by such scientific[xxxvii] experts as Vladimir Janda and as well as Punjabi and White. For those seeking more detailed anatomic information visit **www.bodyzone.com\muscleanatomy** and **www.bodyzone.com\braincontrol.**

INJURY

Pain Cycles begin with an injury. Injuries can be from something big—a macro-trauma—or the accumulation of many little things, called micro-traumas.

A **macro-trauma** is a significant injury or accident that strains tissues past their capacity to stretch. Suddenly twisting and spraining your right knee while running because you are unconsciously leaning to the right is a macro-trauma. When the strength of the tissue is exceeded, its fibers tear. Automobile accidents, sports injuries, and other traumas place a tissue under greater stress than it is designed for, and something gives. Sometimes only a few fibers of a muscle or ligament are damaged, and they can heal uneventfully. Other times there are significant amounts of tissue torn and as a result permanent scarring occurs. But, generally speaking, you know if there has been a macro-trauma. Something happens and it hurts.

Many times muscle and joint macro-traumas occur without a "good" reason. For example, I have seen many patients suffer a "back attack." This kind of sudden, severe pain injury occurs when opposing muscles that should be working smoothly together "miss a beat" and don't properly coordinate, overloading a weak link of the kinetic chain. The overstress may focus on a muscle, ligament, or tendon, or most likely some combination of tissues, but something gives or tears. Much of the positive reputation chiropractic enjoys comes from the almost instant pain relief some of these patients experience when an adjustment realigns the buckled joints to reduce stress on the ligaments and muscles (as well as possibly reducing nerve compression).

On the other hand, a **micro-trauma** is the subtler but equally real injury that occurs when part of the body is subjected to more stress over time than it can handle[xxxviii]. Any mechanical system, be it a bridge or a body, can fail from either dramatically too much stress at one time (macro-trauma), or from much less stress over a long period of time (micro-trauma).

Just as an engineer building a bridge will rate a steel beam to hold X number of tons, the body's muscles and joints are designed to withstand a certain amount of stress. If there is a sign saying "No Trucks Over 15,000 lbs," the bridge will most likely not fall down if you drove a 25,000-lb truck over it. However, if it were hundreds of such trucks each day, we would not be surprised to see the bridge fall down sooner or later. And while metal is not flesh, both will weaken and ultimately fail when overstressed.

Micro-trauma is the failure of body tissues that gradually occurs when over time they are forced to carry more than the capacity for which they were designed. The human frame is a mechanical system, and when the body is used in ways that cause excessive stress on muscles and joints, there's wear on the body's moving parts. This kind of mechanical stress can begin as little injuries from everyday mechanical use and abuse, and frequently doesn't cause immediate pain, but breakdown does occur with time.

Micro-trauma includes the many back problems with their root in prolonged sitting[xxxix], when the normally elastic muscles, tendons, and ligaments are kept under stress so that they lose some of their rebound. Called "elastic creep," like a stretched out rubber band, this loss of rebound in spinal ligaments causes a loss of stability and predisposes the back to injury from motions that would otherwise not be a problem.

Micro-trauma also occurs in the patient with longstanding postural distortions. The man whose posture leans to the right and who complains of a generalized knee pain that began with "no apparent reason" may be suffering from the daily stress on knee ligaments. Or the patient with a softball injury to her ankle may limp to avoid pain, but in so doing stress her other ankle, knee, or low back. When an individual reflexively tightens (and hence over-uses) some muscles to protect and avoid (and hence under-use) other muscles, the body learns to move differently. Even after the injury is healed, the effects of the adaptation persist. And with time, the pain may go away, but the changed pattern of motion doesn't.

Micro-trauma injury can be subtle, resulting from sitting, poor posture, and other habits of life. The silent effects of changed motion patterns is one reason some researchers, such as Gordon Wadell, believe the injury model of low back pain is obsolete and that routine back pain is usually not attributable to a discrete injury or specific injured structure[xl]. The hairdresser who holds his hands up cutting hair all day, the computer operator typing all day, the factory worker moving boxes from left to right (but not from right to left), or the mom carrying her child only on her left hip all stress their body in an asymmetrical way, causing uneven stress and wear.

Whether micro- or macro-trauma, we usually first address an injury for one simple reason: **PAIN.**

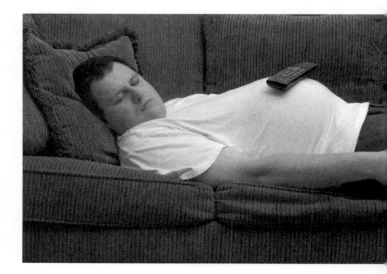

▲ **Figure 7-7** Poor posture habits cause micro-trauma leading to neck and back pain.

PAIN

> *"A quarter of American adults experienced back pain for a full day during the past month.*
> *1 in 10 reports pain lasting a year or more.*
> *Lower back pain is among the most common complaints, along with joint pain, aching or stiffness.*
> Centers for Disease Control, November 2006[xli]

No one likes pain. Despite the aberrant proclivities of some I've heard about, I never met anyone who considers bashing their finger in a car door a good time. And while there may be benefits from being in pain both social (e.g., my back is hurting so I can't mow the lawn and I need to rest on the couch so I may as well watch the game) and psychological (e.g., I am loved because you are caring for me), the actual experience of pain is unpleasant.

But when you stop and think about it, pain is a funny thing. It's commonly said that you can't remember the actual feeling of pain, only that it did hurt, and that you didn't like it. Also, believe it or not, pain is your body's friend. It tells you when tissue is being damaged, so you can react appropriately, say by taking your hand off a hot stove, pain is not always a bad thing and it is important to differentiate between good and bad pain. If you have not exercised, and you use a muscle, it may be sore. Not pleasant perhaps, but not a bad thing. There may be pain, possibly considerable pain, when a professional performs some deep massage on a muscle in spasm, unlocks a trigger point, or does an assisted stretch on a long-restricted joint as in Action Release™ or Graston™ techniques. However, you know it is a good thing afterward when you feel better, and enjoy a greater freedom of motion. On the other hand, the pain that occurs if someone is massaging a joint that is swollen, or stretches a joint in a direction that increases the strain, or further damages an injured tissue, is not good, and should obviously be avoided. The challenge becomes telling the good pain from the bad.

There are two clinical main categories of pain: acute and chronic pain.

Acute pain is when something happens, it hurts, and then it gets better.

Chronic pain is when the pain doesn't fully leave and continues, or recurs periodically, especially from doing activities that should not cause a problem.

This often happens when an acute injury is never allowed to fully heal, and as a result the tissues are weak, allowing subsequent re-injury to the same area.

Some people say they can take a lot of pain; others react strongly to the possibility of pain even if no actual pain has occurred. Many people have taught themselves to "live with the pain" and many consider it a badge of character to be able to "keep on going" despite pain. In fact, living with pain can actually train the body to hurt[xlii] as the Contracting, Connecting, and Control motion systems interact and reinforce patterns of pain and motion.

> Disorders such as reflex sympathetic dystrophy (RSD) can occur when someone's nerves become so sensitive to pain that their ability to transmit pain information along those paths is increased a hundredfold, and what would otherwise be a slight discomfort becomes an agonizing episode.

However, far more common than neurological pain disorders are the millions of people experiencing, and living with, everyday "normal" pain. In the absence of illness, **pain is not normal**.

However, in addition to being a common factor in the Pain Cycle, living in pain can have dramatic consequences.

> Chronic low back pain has been shown to cause premature brain aging. Over the course of a 1-year study of chronic pain sufferers, MRIs showed 10-20 times more loss of gray matter than in normal control subjects[xliii].

Chronic pain and poor posture are the accumulation of old injuries on our LifeHabits as our bodies adapt to pain. We are not talking about grimacing pain, or pain that causes one to cry out, but low-grade, constant, you-can't-get-away-from-it pain. The kind of pain that makes you stop doing the things in life you used to, or want to, enjoy. The kind of pain that many people think is "normal," as you stop doing, and live with it.

If it hurts to move, the body will compensate and move in a way to avoid pain.

148|

COMPENSATION

People will move however they can to avoid pain. If it hurts to stand or sit, we instinctively change our posture. Short term this is normal, and not a problem. It becomes a problem when you become comfortable with it.

The unbalanced motion from an injury, or even habitual poor posture, causes muscular imbalance. As some muscles strengthen to meet the demands of the uneven load, other muscles shorten and weaken. Overall the body compensates, causing balance, alignment, and motion to change.

Body motion should be symmetrical—the head should turn as far to the left as the right[xliv]. So, when there is asymmetric, uneven motion, even if someone believes they are moving normally, the body must compensate. Therefore, any asymmetric restriction of motion must result in a change in motion, a compensation.

Changes in Contracting, Connecting, and Control systems all interact to maintain balance, or gravity wins and we fall down. Compensation is three dimensional. Nerves learn patterns to control muscles that strengthen *specifically* in the ways they move joints, whose motion is restricted by restraining ligaments that have shortened or stretched.

Clinically, we frequently see patients with a history of multiple problems. Like the layers of an onion, as current symptoms are resolved previously hidden adaptations and pains may resurface in a process called retracing.

I had a patient who initially complained of right shoulder pain when playing tennis. He also reported having had a history of low back pain, but being OK for the past two years or so. After assessing a motion problem in the neck and shoulder (shoulder muscles attach to the neck and nerves from the neck control the shoulder), we treated him with good results. However, a few weeks later he came back, reporting a recurrence of low back pain. When he asked if fixing his shoulder could have stressed his back, I countered by asking him what brought up that question. His answer: "It feels like since you fixed my shoulder I am moving the way I did when my back hurt."

In all candor, my leaning is he was correct— his shoulder was being stressed because of asymmetric

motion to compensate for his low back problem. So when I adjusted his neck and shoulder to encourage symmetrical motion, the compensation for his low back problem was once again stressed. We then successfully treated the low back with manipulations and focused StrongPosture™ exercises.

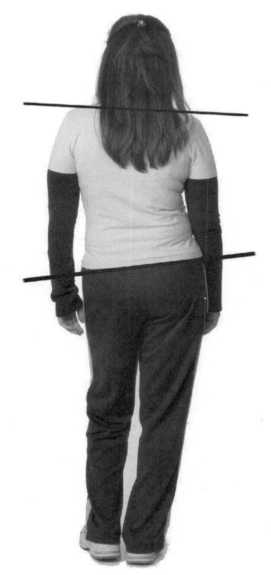

▲ **Figure 7-8** Shoulder-pelvis posture compensation

Compensation can be psychological as well as physical[xlv]. People actually get used to living with pain. Also, when someone takes pain medication on a frequent or even daily basis to cover up chronic pain, they come to believe the pain, as well as the regular drug use, is normal.

> Chronic low back pain sufferers are especially at risk for what psychologists call "fear avoidance behavior[xlvi]". Someone who experiences anxiety from anticipating pain and thus avoids activity ranging from exercise to work has a psychosocial problem as well as a physical one, placing them at increased risk for disability[xlvii]. The Pain Cycle spirals larger with inactivity; immobilization; and disuse; tissue impairment leading to reduced strength and range of motion; stiffness; weakness; reduced motor skills, balance, and stability; and increased risk of injury, which leads to more fear avoidance. Experts, such as Liebenson, recommend restoring motion slowly, reassuring the patient to progressively increase function and to differentiate the good pain of restored joint and muscle function from the bad pain of tissue damage.

Regardless of the psychological aspect, when there is injury and tissue damage, there is pain. The pain then causes the body to compensate and move in a way to avoid pain. And as we will see, over time layers of subsequent adaptations occur because of real, physical changes in the Contracting, Connecting, and Control systems.

Compensation and Muscles (Contracting system)

If you have ever had a back problem, you quickly observed it hurt to move "like this," but it felt better to move "like that." We are hardwired to avoid pain so you move in whatever way you can find that doesn't hurt. The problem is, muscles strengthen **specifically** as they are used.

Muscles connect bones, and contract to either move OR stabilize a joint. For example, our body would tumble to the ground if it weren't for opposing muscles simultaneously contracting to stiffen the joints on which we balance. The spine is the mast of the body, and is stabilized by spinal muscles working together so it can carry twenty times the load that its ligaments alone could carry without buckling[xlviii].

If you recall when we talked about muscles, the muscle cell is either fully contracted or not contracted at all. This all-or-none effect means when you move differently you strengthen some while other muscle fibers that should normally be working get weaker. Asymmetric motion creates patterns of muscle motion by strengthening muscles specifically. We'll discuss more about adaptation and muscles in the 5th Posture Principle.

Compensation and Ligaments, etc.
(Connecting system)

Ligaments are like rubber bands that hold bones together passively, or without effort. But unbalanced and asymmetric motion keeps some joints in a narrow range of motion, shortening ligaments.

> After only twenty minutes of sitting, some spinal ligaments will shorten as the fibers rearrange because of elastic creep. And as people whose backs stiffen after sitting know, even after changing posture the ligaments do not fully lengthen for some time[xlix].

The Connecting system responds to both macro- and micro-injury and trauma, and it may only heal with 50% of its strength even six months after injury and 80% after one year. Depending upon the stresses and new injuries it endures in daily life, it may take up to three years for the ligament to get back to 100%[l]. In fact, some researchers argue that if a muscle or ligament injury is not completely healed within six weeks, damage to blood supply[li] and mechanical adaptation become permanent, resulting in a chronic problem[lii]. So if an injury ever made you limp, or otherwise move differently for more than a week or so, you probably have some scar tissue or adhesions that even now, in the absence of pain, cause your posture and motion to continue to "give" to that old injury.

NOTE: Also, all the motion systems—Connecting, Contracting and Control—begin healing from injury with inflammation, which causes pain, reduces motion with swelling to prevent further damage, and creates a "stickiness" that can cause adhesions and promote scar tissue, further limiting the ability to move fully and freely.

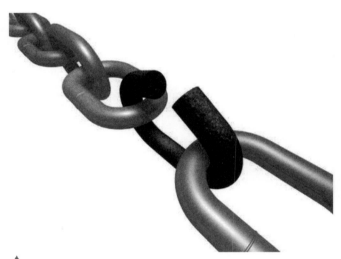

▲ **Figure 7-9** A chain of motion is only as strong as the weakest link

Compensation and the Brain, Nerves and Receptors (Control System)

Just as the muscles of the Contracting system strengthens and the Connecting ligaments stretch as they're stressed, the Control system get better at working in the ways they are used. Just as a used muscle trains and becomes stronger, nerves become trained to better transmit information. Like a well-traveled path in the woods, the 4th Posture Principle means your body learns what you teach it as often-utilized nerve pathways become easier for the body to use in a process scientists call facilitation.

There is a saying in neurology, "Nerves that fire together, wire together." The concept is called neuroplasticity, which is a fancy way of saying that nerves learn, and nerve pathways get better at transmitting whatever information you train them to send.

Sensory Nerve Compensation

Some nerves are incoming, and carry information into the brain from the body. Others are outgoing, carrying information out from the brain to the body.

> The constant stream of traffic between the brain and the body travels on one-way lanes composed of two unique types of nerves: incoming sensory (or afferents) and outgoing motor (or efferents).

Not only do both kinds of nerves get better at transmitting their unique messages, but the brain itself gets better at how it processes, senses, and reacts to the information it receives.

> The five senses we learned in grade school—sight, hearing, smell, taste, and touch—also send information to the brain on unique pathways. We don't hear on smell nerves or taste on sight nerves. Called tracts as they travel through the brain, these nerve highways are the wires, each sending a different kind of information, as each part of the brain and spinal cord learns to do what it does better with use.

> For example, the taste buds and sense of smell of a wine connoisseur are more sensitive than mine because of hours spent using those nerves, and strengthening those nerve pathways. On the other hand, I am a chiropractor, and in school they taught me to develop my sense of touch so I can palpate someone's joint to detect tension and swelling an untrained hand could not. (By the way, that is how chiropractors "know" where it hurts...we are trained to feel for the tissue changes that accompany pain.)

Pain information is transmitted by specific kinds of nerves, and just as muscles and other nerves get better at doing what they do, pain nerves get better at transmitting the message "It hurts." I find the kind of pride some people show about "living with pain" ironic because they are frequently actually training their body to hurt.

> Injury not only causes pain, but causes pain nerves to stimulate larger numbers of other pain-sensing nerves within the spinal cord[liii].

From a doctor's point of view, the patient with acute pain from an injury is easier to care for. The patient and doctor both expect it to get better in short order. Far more frustrating is chronic pain that doesn't go away. Current research shows that another big part of the problem literally comes from having had pain. Nerves get better at doing what they are trained to do, including feeling pain.

> Studies of neuropathic pain (deep, unrelenting, nerve-based pain) show it is the healthy nerve fibers, not the injured ones, that are sending the pain messages to the brain[liv].

Some researchers argue that problems such as chronic back pain can occur for no other reason than the person has been hurting! If this sounds like a circular reasoning, it is—but it can be true.

> *"Pain may be due to disturbed function without any structural damage. You do not need structural damage to have pain from musculoskeletal dysfunction."* Gordon Waddell, MD. The Back Pain Revolution[lv].

Motor Nerve Compensation

Motor nerves are lanes for the outgoing traffic telling muscle to contract. As discussed earlier, muscle memory (or neuromuscular memory) occurs not solely from changes in muscle, but primarily from nerves getting better at transmitting information. And since the contraction of each individual muscle cell is controlled by commands from motor nerves, we get better at doing whatever we do very specifically.

Some people talk about negative or positive muscle memory. However, even though mechanical stress or effectiveness may be lesser or greater, there are no value judgments in how we learn to move. The body simply learns to do whatever you teach it (within its physical capacity, of course). The point is, the body learns motions without regard to whether they are good or bad—like water cutting a path in the dirt, which becomes a stream and then a river, motion simply follows the path of least resistance and the Contracting, Connecting, and Control systems get better at doing what they do.

Compensation in the Brain and Spinal Cord

Our brain is an amazing 3-pound organ that collects and correlates incoming sense information and then sends out signals to control muscles with split second precision. But the incoming information consists of more than the five senses.

> For example, touch is really four different senses because four different sets of nerves send the brain information about heat, cold, pressure, and pain.

Experts argue about the number of internal senses (Is hunger or sexual desire a sense? Is the sense of direction internal or is it the result of thinking about information you have already sensed?), but all agree on the importance of balance and proprioception, the kinesthetic senses, for posture and body motion.

Researchers are constantly learning how nerve functions, as well as our perceptions, are more complex than was believed even a few years ago[lvi, lvii]. Much of our reaction to signals (such as pain) is programmed into our bodies; some of it is learned, and all of it occurs from the brain and spinal cord nerves ultimately connecting incoming sensory and outgoing motor signals. The brain has been compared to a computer made of nerve cells with built-in programs, as well as the ability to create new programs, our physical experiences and injury as well as both conscious and unconscious intentions, actions, and decisions all shape these programs as we continually get better at doing whatever we do.

The controlling nervous systems of creatures from white mice to humans learn when nerve pathways get better at transmitting the information they are designed to transmit. The first time a child touches a hot stove, it may take a moment for them to pull their hand away. But today, if you unwittingly put you hand on a hot stove, you will reflexively pull it off, usually before you actually perceive much pain. The perception and anticipation of pain can cause other changes and reactions in the body such as your heart racing in an adrenaline surge. And the next time you come close to touching a hot stove, you will pull away a tad more quickly.

Patterns of motion control posture and the body, and are learned. Pain channels us away from some patterns and into others, creating motor amnesias and resulting in muscle weakness, imbalance, and ultimately loss of ability to move in unused patterns.

»TRY THIS: *Morning Freeze*

We learned in the 2nd Posture Principle, Balance, about how far-from-fully understood connections deep within the brain integrate information from the visual, the vestibular, and the proprioceptive systems to balance posture and control our body in space. The kinesthetic sense is how we know where we are in space.

Try this: When you wake up tomorrow morning, **DON'T MOVE**. Then, try to be aware of where your right leg is compared to your left leg **WITHOUT MOVING YOUR BODY**.
You may find you have "body amnesia" until you move the leg. Moving the leg stimulates the motor and joint receptors that tell the brain where the body is in space.

Also note: What position are your hands in? Your arms?

»TRY THIS: *The Hand Roll*

The hand roll demonstrates the challenge of control and coordination.

Rotate your left hand in a circle. Then rotate it toward you. No problem, right?

Now, rotate your right hand away from you. Still easy? **Simultaneously, rotate your left hand toward you.**

Can't? Here's why.

You probably noticed your motion pattern is either both hands away OR both hands toward you. Like rubbing your belly and patting your head, unless trained otherwise, we keep on moving in familiar patterns.

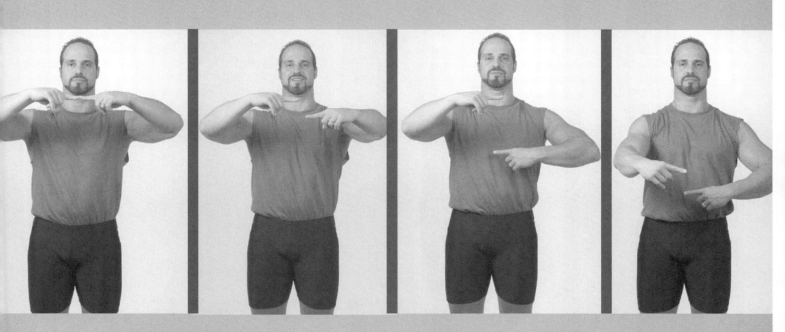

▲ **Figure 7-10** HandRoll A,B,C

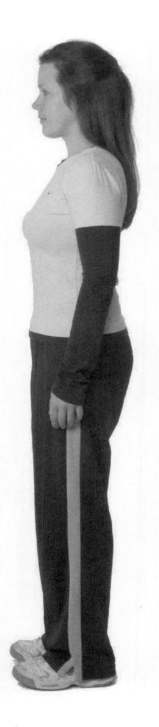
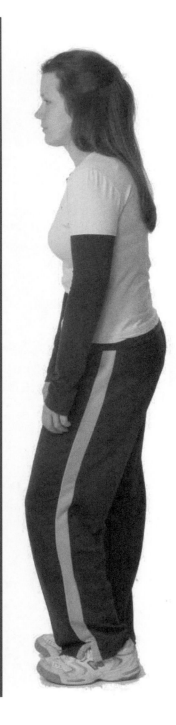

Unbalanced Motion
...and Posture
...and Motion

The brain is constantly receiving vital posture information. You may not be conscious of this posture control information, but you depend on it in whenever you move your body. Strong (or weak) posture and balance depends on the alignment between where the brain perceives our body to be and where the body truly is.

Everyone has a subtle, complex, and unconscious perception of his or her own body. When you have pain and limitation of motion due to an injury, you adapt your body image to fit that limitation. This unconscious mental adaptation often persists long after the injury has been resolved in the way we move and even breathe.

The kinesthetic sense of proprioception sends information about where our body is in space, how much tension there is on this muscle or that tendon, and in which direction and how quickly a part of our body is moving in relation to a different part. If you think your head is over your feet, and you are wrong, your balance is weak because to stay upright you must unconsciously use other muscles to compensate.

◀ **Figure 7-11** Strong vs. weak posture

»TRY THIS: *Standing Balance Compensation Test*

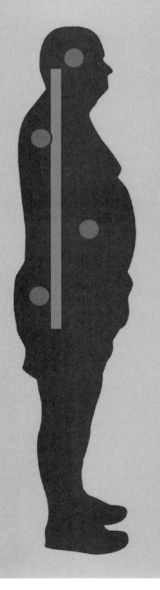

Focus on your posture.
Now, stand holding one part of your body differently (e.g., put your hip out to the left)
Notice: You must do more than one thing differently (i.e., shift your shoulders to the right) to balance or you will fall down.

Compensating for posture begins a cascade of changes. Muscles and joints compensate for lost motion in one part of the kinetic chain, which then affects others because all must work together to balance. When posture has compensated, physiologic changes in all three motion systems—Control, Connecting, and Contracting— and set a new baseline for posture, affecting how we move in everyday life, reducing the effectiveness of exercise and limiting athletic performance.

Unbalanced MOTION leads to

INEFFECTIVE EXERCISE

Practice doesn't make perfect...practice make permanent.

Figure 7-12 Poor posture affects performance and how we move

156|

Compensating for Compensation with
StrongPosture™ Exercise

If you exercise lopsided, your body develops lopsided. Over time, unbalanced motion causes actual changes as the body adapts, which brings us to the 5th and final Posture principle, **ADAPTATION**. But before we go into how adaptation can either make us move old or give us a tool to move young, let's progress with our StrongPosture™ exercises and learn to stabilize the torso, open the chest, and strengthen pelvic control.

Stronger Breathing

We learned earlier how breathing is the body-mind link. Now that you have been doing StrongPosture™ exercises for a few days, see if you find new motions when doing these focused breathing exercises.

> *Conscious Breathing and WallTilts Focus*
> Conscious breathing focuses StrongPosture™ exercise to control unused muscles.
> > Do WallTilt and breathe in *as slowly as you possibly can,* taking in as deep a breath as you can.
> > > Coordinate your breathing with the slow motion of your pelvic arch

> *Notice: Are you breathing with your Belly or Chest?*

Strong breathing uses your diaphragm, a sheet of muscle separating the lungs in the chest from the abdomen. This sheet begins at a critical biomechanical point on the front of the spine, where the fibers of the diaphragm are intertwined with those of another main posture muscle, the hip flexors, or psoas.

> If you place your hand behind your mid-back (just below where a woman's bra-strap would be) and breathe in deeply, you can feel the spine move with your breath.

Clinically this explains the often profound effect of psoas as well as diaphragm therapy and exercise on posture. Body motion is a chain following the path of least resistance, so restriction of either the psoas or the diaphragm affects the other muscle.

> A common problem with teaching some people to do pelvic tilts is that they stop breathing. Then when cued to breathe, they stop moving the pelvis and begin moving their chest. Especially common in people suffering with mid-back tension and pain, they can often get tremendous relief once they learn to separate the motion of their pelvis and their breath.

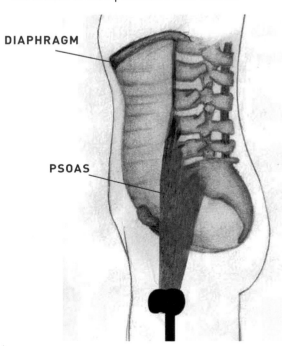

DIAPHRAGM

PSOAS

▲ **Figure 7-13** Diaphragm-psoas anatomy

Try taking 5 breaths doing these focuses to become aware of your breathing pattern and strengthening your control.

Hands-on-Ribs Breathing

1. Put your hands on the sides of the ribs.
2. Breathe in and expand your ribs out against your hands.
3. Breathe out and gently push in your ribs to fully exhale
4. Repeat for 5 slow breaths. Stop if you feel dizzy or light-headed.

Towel Crisscross

Crisscross a towel or scarf around your torso, holding a towel end in each hand.
As you breathe in keep a gentle tension on the towel.
Try to feel where you are breathing from.
Now, try to focus your breath into your sides.
> As you inhale, try to feel your lower ribs expand. Keep your chest quiet, and shift motion from your belly to your sides and back.

Repeat for five slow breaths.

Breathing Visualizations

1. Imagine your belly is a big balloon:
> Each time you inhale, fill the balloon. Feel the expansion all the way down into deepest part of your lower pelvis and all the way up through your neck. Keep your shoulders relaxed.
2. Imagine there is a big balloon behind your low back
> Fill it up as you arch, and push the air out of it as you tuck.

Advanced Breathing Exercises

(1) Exhale Bias Breath
> Try to breathe in for a count of 8, and then out for a count of 4.

(2) Inhale Bias Breath
> Try to breathe in for a count of 4, and then out for a count of 8.

(3) Balanced Breath
> Try to breathe in for a count of 6, and then out for a count of 6.

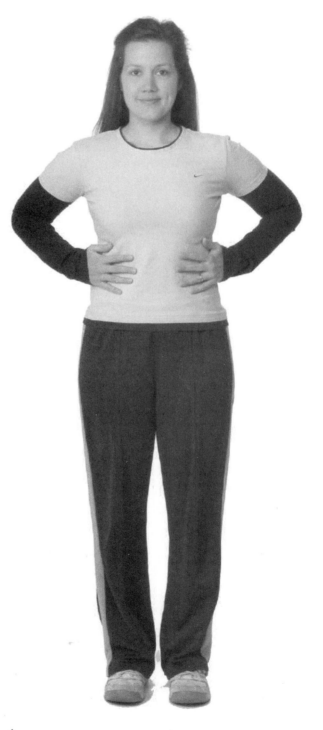

▲ **Figure 7-14** Hands-on-ribs breathing

StrongPosture™ Alignment:
Arms UP
Shoulder Girdle Stabilization with Strong Breath WallTilts

Arm Positioning and Shoulder Blade retraction with pelvic tilt

Forward head posture and forward rolled shoulders are common problems in our sitting society. Arms UP pelvic tilts give you an anytime stretch and exercise to help relieve neck and upper back stress.

Goal: Train coordination of shoulder position while doing a pelvic tilt with neck retraction to strengthen neglected shoulder girdle stabilizing muscles.

The Exercise

Begin by doing a WallTilt.
> Focus on keeping your arms flat against the wall
> Imagine bungee cords pulling your middle finger out toward the floor.

Breathe in and arch, and
> Press the back of your hands and arms into the wall, keeping them there as you tuck.

Breathe out and tuck,

Try to make the tips of the shoulder blades touch, keeping them there as you tuck.

Breathe in and arch, and
> With controlled motion, lift your Arms UP so they are at 90 degrees to your body.

Breathe out and tuck, keep your head, shoulders and arms strong and stable.
> Keep your neck strong retracted and keep your:
>> Shoulders and head level
>> Shoulders down
>> Elbows bent to 90 degrees
>> Palms aligned with the forearm and wrists straight

Keep StrongPosture™!

> Touch elbows to wall
> Touch hands to wall
> Point fingers to ceiling

Continue doing WallTilts, counting with 5 slow breaths
> Keep the head level and retracted with shoulders down and upper arms stable
> Keep shoulders against wall and elbows against the wall
> Keep the hand aligned with the wrist

Try to:
> Press elbow to wall
> Press hands to wall
> Pull the tips of the shoulder blades together.

▼ **Figure 7-15** Arms UP with WallTilt

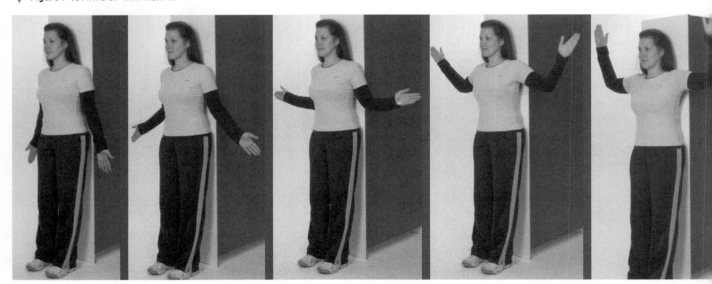

StrongPosture™ Motion:
BallHug

Purpose: Unlock restricted vertebral joints

The BallHug relaxes spinal muscles and helps relieve pain by de-stressing the spinal joints, fully opening the joints and allowing spinal muscles to lengthen. Our goal is to build a 5-minute Strong Motion exercise routine on the ball that flows together, one into the other. We'll be adding SideStretch later to connect BallSit-BackStretch-Abfocus with BallHug before continuing into controlled torso extension with Superman.

Goal: Spinal relaxation and flexion (passive)

AWARE POSITION: On your stomach hugging the ball

CONTROLLED MOTION: Hug the ball. Roll forward and backward, allowing the spine to stretch.

BREATHING FLOW: Relax and roll your torso over ball.
    Keep your neck retracted to lengthen your neck
    Do a pelvic tilt or two to unlock your pelvis
Stretch for 5 slow, controlled breaths

▼ **Figure 7-16** BallHug

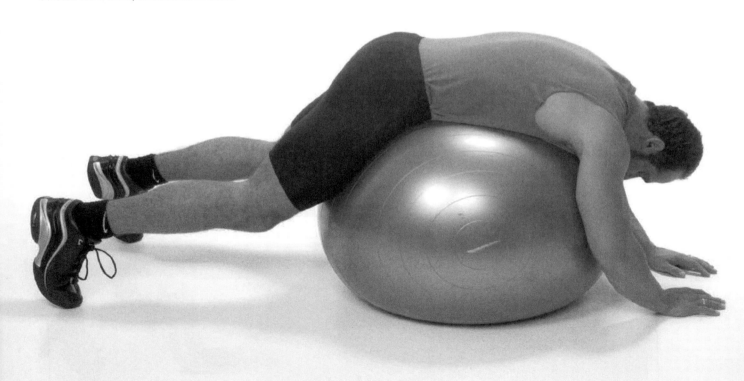

160|

SideStretch BallHug Transition

The goal of a daily StrongPosture™ exercise is training control with coordinated motion.

GOAL: Connect face up and face down ball exercises using core muscles to smoothly move from AbFocus to SideStretch to BallHug.

AWARE POSITION: From SideStretch, step over your leg and use controlled motion to roll over into BallHug.

Do a pelvic tilt to stabilize the pelvis

Move with control

If you roll past your stomach, bounce out of control or are otherwise moving by "flinging" your body, try to focus on pulling your belly button in to activate your core muscles and effectively stabilize.

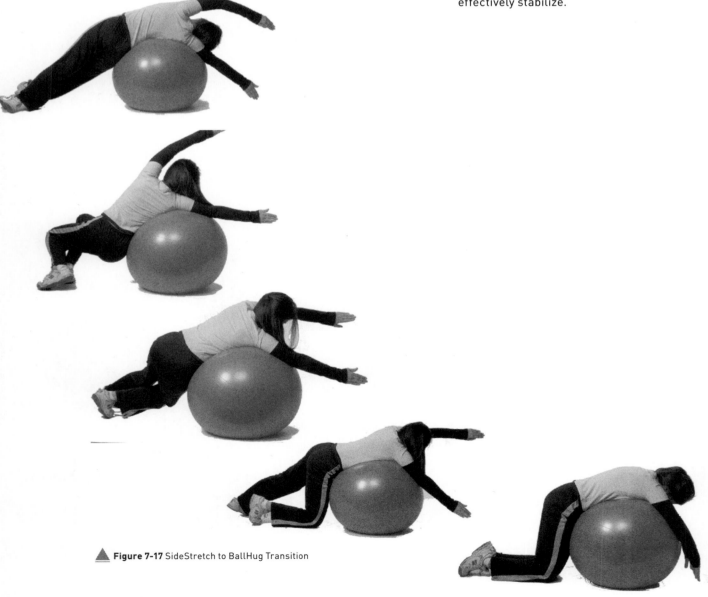

▲ **Figure 7-17** SideStretch to BallHug Transition

StrongPosture™
7 Week Program-

B
A
M

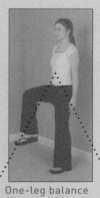

One-leg balance
(**The Stork**)-p.19

Strong Balance

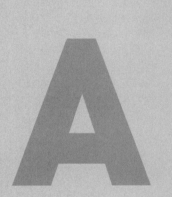

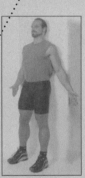

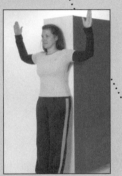

WallTilt -p66   **ArmsUp** -p.158

Strong Alignment

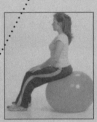

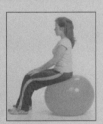

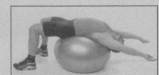

BallStretch -p.101

BallTilt Arch -p.75   **BallTilt Tuck** -p.75

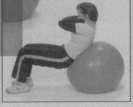

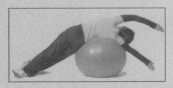

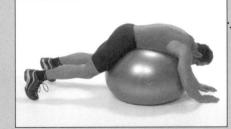

AbFocus -p.131   **SideStretch** -p.103   **BallHug** -p.159

Strong Motion

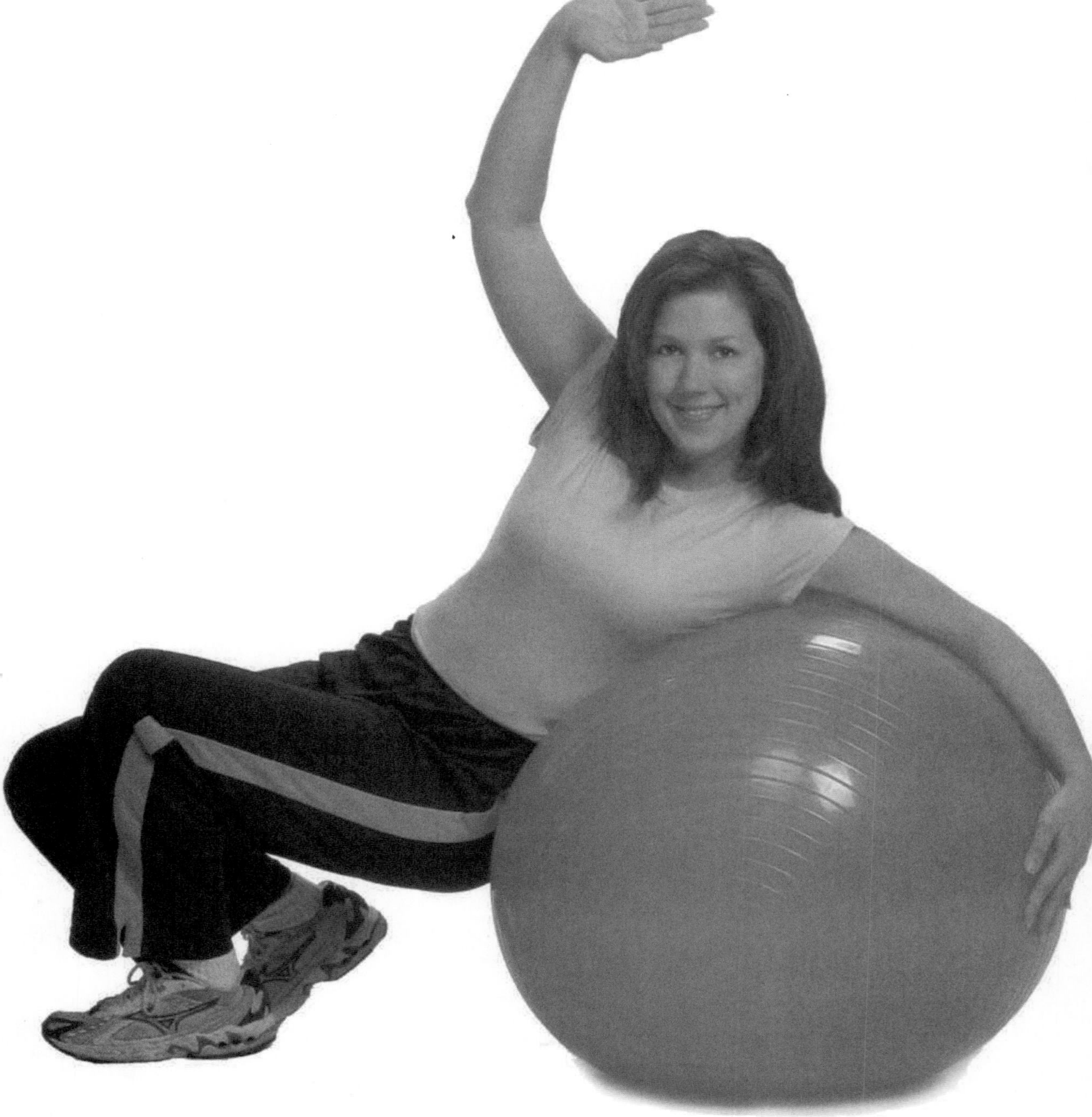

8 Adaptation
The 5th Posture Principle

Changes in Posture & Motion
Cause the Body to Change

. . . for worse, or for better

*"It's not the things we know that gets us in trouble.
It's the things we know that ain't so."* Artemus Ward

The 5th and final Posture Principle, Adaptation, together with the first four principles, shows how, for better or for worse, our posture LifeHabits literally change our body over time.

Motion is the 1st Posture Principle and deals with the architecture, structure, and biology of how we move. Balance, the 2nd, deals with how we keep our body upright.

The 3rd Posture Principle concerns the Patterns arising from the interaction of the first two principles. Compensation, the 4th principle, ties the first three together to explain how your body moves differently to best navigate the path between pain and the capabilities of each link in the chain. Adaptation is the 5th principle, and focuses on changes in structure from Compensation.

We know posture and balance are two sides of the same coin, and that it's not just your posture but how you balance the body (including the relative motions of all the different weight-bearing joints) that determines how your body moves. Similarly, compensation and adaptation are intimately related concepts that together explain the effects of posture on performance as well as on pain and aging. StrongPosture™ means you're more stable and have better control so performance improves and you suffer fewer injuries. Not only is the golfer who can't bend over straight to pick up a ball avoiding pain by twisting to the side as he bends, he is training both a bad shot and a bad back.

Hunched over "old posture" and other postural changes we associate with aging occur from the spiraling effects of compensation and adaptation to our postural environment. From a postural point of view, environment refers to where your body physically is and what it's doing.

Any set of positions and motions that the body inhabits for a significant period of time is a postural environment. It may be an occasional physical activity such as golf or tennis; an everyday physical activity like hammering nails or typing on a computer; or it may be a pervasive sedentary activity such as driving, watching TV, playing a videogame, or reading a book.

Postural aging is a vicious cycle of compensating for our environment, then physically adapting to optimize function within that environment, which then changes how the body moves and balances, resulting in more compensation, followed by more adaptation, in an ever-tightening spiral toward a geriatric walker.

> *In a self-regulating mechanism, such as the human body, adaptation and compensation to such structural changes takes place, but always at the expense of optimum, or perfect, function. Such alterations in function may remain within acceptable limits, and not produce noticeable symptoms, but as will be seen, if these changes occur in vital spinal areas, widespread effects may take place, distant from the area of dysfunction. Structure and function should not be thought of as separate entities, one is inconceivable without the other*[lviii].
> Leon Chaitow, Principles of Osteopathy

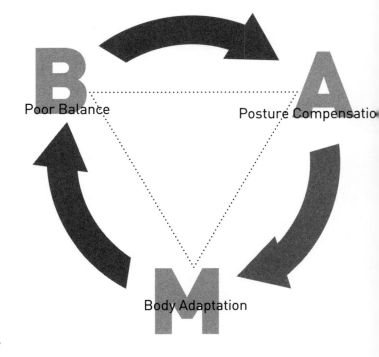

▲ **Figure 8-1** Compensation- Adaptation- Balance spiral

Posture Breakdown:
How changes in motion cause changes for the worse in our Contracting, Connecting, and Control systems

"Most musculoskeletal pain and dysfunction results from the failure of adaptation, where self-regulation compensation mechanisms reach a point of exhaustion, so that de-compensation eventuates. " Hans Selye, noted scientist and originator of the concept that stress is a diseaselix.

The Insidious Problem of Our Sitting Society

There are 3 D's of Posture Degeneration:

- DNA -The genetics you are born with and cannot change.

- Damage to your body, from injuries both recalled and forgotten, which can be avoided, but the history of injury cannot be erased.

- Daily LifeHabits, or how you use and move your body every day.

Lack of motion of specific joints in specific directions is the common thread connecting problems of sitting and posture. People use tools (yes, a chair is a tool) to change how we live, and in turn our bodies change as we adapt and compensate.

This compensation affects the body's mechanics because we still have to balance, affecting the relative alignment, strength, and flexibility of the posture's kinetic chain of motion, including:

Foot, knee, and leg and hip alignment

Pelvic position (tilted forward, back, or to either side)

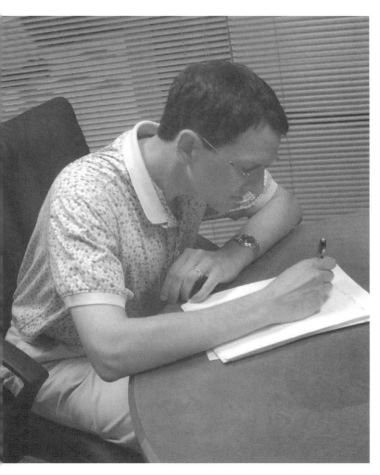

Figure 8-2 Sitting is the 21ˢᵗ century posture

166|

and abdominal protrusion

Lumbar spine alignment and curve, stressing discs in the low back

Thoracic spine alignment and curve, stressing discs in the upper back

Cervical spine alignment and curve, stressing discs in the **neck**

The position of the head in relation to the shoulders

The shoulder girdle and rotator cuff

The relative position and motion of the arms, elbows, and hands

The possible combinations of motion are very large. However, once body motions compensate for pain, some motions get stronger and others get weaker as the body adapts. Changes to the Contracting, Connecting and Control systems train the new pattern of motion, and over time new injuries and problems cause progressively more adaptations, resulting in adaptive possibilities being used up.

■ If you can't lift your arm over your head due to a shoulder injury, you will compensate by over-arching your lower back when you reach overhead.

■ If your left knee hurts, you will lean to the right to ease the pain as you walk, and so also overwork your right-side low back muscles and left-side upper back muscles.

■ If your feet pronate (roll in), or if you are flat-footed, pigeon-toed, or have one leg shorter than another, your posture will shift as you distort your pelvis and spine to stand up.

Like a mouse in a maze, we move adaptively to run away from pain, but ultimately as we lose options from a pain-free repertoire of full motion, we end up with no place to move without pain. Fewer and fewer possibilities of motion continually restrict us from comfortable positions and our overall motion becomes restricted and irregular.

The old person shuffling along suffering from decreasing complexity of motion along with weakened balance is

demonstrating two cardinal signs of age-related posture degeneration[ix]. Add on the accumulation of Pain Cycle injuries from the body constantly adapting to weak balance and it's easy to see why people so often associate posture degeneration with "normal aging." For better or for worse, our Contracting, Connecting and Control systems all adapt.

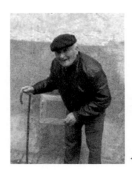

Figure 8-3 Spinal stress causes changes

Aging poorly = Stiffness + weakness =

Inability to move normally = Loss of function

Adaptation and the Connecting System-Ligaments, Joints, Tendons, and Fascia

> *Wolff's Law*
> *The principle that every change in the form and the function of a bone or in the function of the bone alone, leads to changes in its internal architecture and in its external form.*
> The American Heritage® Stedman's Medical Dictionary, 2nd Edition Houghton Mifflin Company 2004

The majority of people over sixty complain of arthritic stiffness and pain in joints ranging from the knees to the hands and from the neck to the toes. The breakdown of Connecting system tissues is aggravated by the common episodic injuries of life escalating through the Pain Cycle, and is blamed for many back problems as well as many of the aches and pains of growing older.

Also known as osteoarthritis or degenerative joint disease (DJD), this common affliction of old age is caused by the mechanical stress of bearing weight and repetitive motion. In addition, injuries damage the inner lining of the joint capsule, affecting its ability to make the fluid lubricating joint motion, further speeding breakdown and accelerating the normal wear and tear of aging. X-rays show thinning of the cartilage that normally protects the bones, and calcium build up (bone spurs) where joint stress occurs, which then irritates the joint capsule and causes pain.

Despite the significance of cartilage breakdown and arthritic deposits as signposts of mechanical stress, there is more to postural pain and degeneration than wear and tear. All the tissues of the body adapt. Someone who is grossly overweight and then loses 100 lbs. will gain weight more easily than someone whose fat cells were not conditioned for efficient storage. Even though we may not think it's fair ("Why can't I have rippling biceps without working out? Why shouldn't I have a second piece of cheesecake?") the tissues of the body get better at doing whatever they are trained to do.

Damage and tears to Connecting system tissues from injury will usually heal. However, problems begin because healing is frequently less than perfect. Scar tissue, adhesions, and

Adaptation and the Contracting System-Muscles

> *"When injured, most tissues heal, but skeletal muscles learn."* Janet Travell, MD

Someone who lifts weights as a teenager will generally strengthen more quickly if they return to lifting weights later in life because the muscle cells have been conditioned, and once conditioned will more easily regain greater function and performance. Muscles strengthen with exercise specifically in the way they are exercised. This basic athletic training concept is called Specific Adaptation of Imposed Demand, or SAID[lxi], and is the reason why weight trainers rotate exercises: if you want to change a body, you have to keep on stressing the body differently. Whether a muscle contracts with a shortening (concentric) contraction or a lengthening (eccentric) contraction, whether it contracts quickly or slowly, the muscle adapts to how it is used and your body learns to do what you teach it (4th Posture Principle).

So, if your goal is moving well as you age, the muscles must be used in the ways today that you want to use them tomorrow.

see www.bodyzone.com/adaptation for more on Adaptation and muscles

other imperfectly healed tissue plus mechanical stress lengthen some fibers and shorten others causing function to change.

> Large or small, adhesions are internal scars fusing muscle, tendon, bursa, or other tissue, thereby limiting freedom of motion. Adhesions can affect areas as small as just a few muscle fibers, or can be spread out throughout a muscle group. Old adhesions limit motion when poorly healed tissues prevent further stretching and cause muscles to reflexively contract to protect the area. Bursitis, tendonitis, and tenosynovitis and other biomechanical problems can result from this mechanical stress. Further changes occur as the body avoids some arcs of motion, causing muscles that do not fully lengthen to lose strength. Also, when even a small segment of a muscle stops contracting, you stress other Connecting system ligaments and tendons that suddenly have to take up the slack. The resulting remodeling of muscles and ligaments begins about three weeks after an injury, and can continue for a year[lxii].

In addition, bones, the architectural framework of the body, also adapt to mechanical stress. Bones can become denser and thicken into a spur, or wear down with microscopic stress fractures.

Just as the uneven stress of a car's misaligned front end (its architecture) will cause its tires to wear unevenly, asymmetrical posture alignment and body motion stresses tissues and causes premature wear. If the tread on your tires is completely worn out on the inside, but still brand new on the outside, you will either buy new tires, or have a blowout. The fact that the outside of your tires is new doesn't help! Just as a chain is only as strong as the weakest link, in the chain of your body's posture and motion, the weak link determines how much you can do, and how long your body will last.

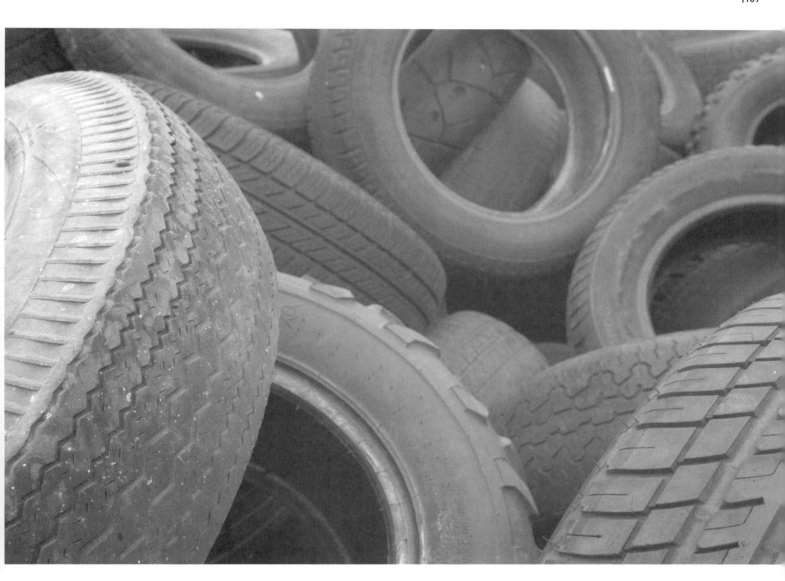

▲ **Figure 8-4** Uneven stress makes tires...and bodies...wear unevenly.

170|

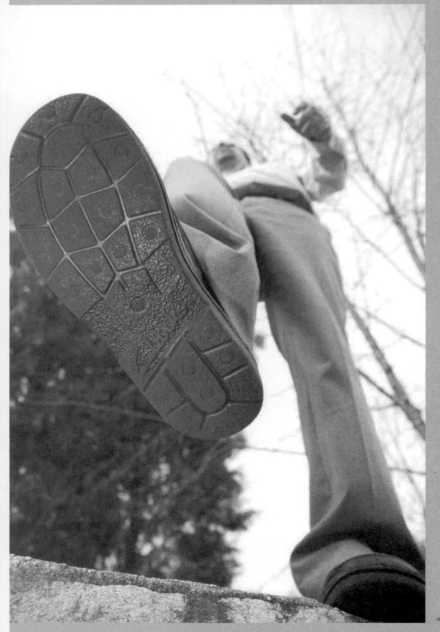

Look at the bottoms and sides of your shoes.
Are they worn the same on both sides?
If not, it is because they have worn to adapt to the stress of your walking unevenly on them. When the tread on the bottom of your shoes wears out unevenly you can buy new shoes.

Where are you going to live when you wear out your body?

Figure 8-5 Sole searching

bad, but which had improved up until a month or so ago, and then again being in bad pain after her dog pulled hard on its leash when she was unprepared.

She brought me the X-rays her MD took, and there was indeed significant arthritic breakdown in the low back and knee joints. However, when I compared them to low back X-rays I had taken five years earlier there was only a very slight difference.

I then asked her if she thought the arthritis had gone away during the time when her pain was gone and then grown back over the past month. She quickly said that was ridiculous. . . which it is.

But. . . if the pain was from the arthritis, and the arthritis is clearly visible on X-ray, if the pain goes away, how can the arthritis be unchanged?

We treated her that day by adjusting her pelvis, knees, and ankle, did some postural therapy, and she reported feeling "80% improved. " About a month later, after a course of adjustments and resuming the StrongPosture™ exercises recommended five years ago, which she had stopped doing (her pain was gone so why keep doing the exercises?), she was back to walking in almost no pain. In addition, she had stopped taking all of the drugs.

Joint damage cannot be reversed, but keeping joints moving and staying active as much as possible can slow further breakdown. Despite bone and cartilage breakdown, stretching tight muscles and fascia can help relieve arthritic pain, as shown in a 2006 study of patients with osteoarthritis of the knee[lxiii].

I have always had a problem with the assertion that arthritis explains any joint problems in people over forty for one reason: almost all of us have some joint problems. . . even if there is no pain whatsoever.

I recently saw a patient whom I had successfully treated for a work-related injury some years ago, and who came in complaining of back and knee pain, which her primary care provider, a medical doctor, had diagnosed as being from arthritis. Over the past six months she reported taking first Advil and then Naprosyn for the pain. In addition, she had just started taking Zantac for her stomach problems, which she and her MD believed was from the other drugs.

She reported having been in pain that was intermittently

Connecting system breakdown from constant, low-grade mechanical stress is a growing problem as evidenced by the dramatic increase in cumulative stress disorders such as Carpal Tunnel Syndrome. Similarly, chronic sitting in a slouched position puts the spinal joints in a flexed position that not only strains the low back, but stretches the ligaments in back and compresses the front cartilage, bending us toward the bent-over posture of an old man.

The engineer who builds bridges knows where stress points occur and so specifies that certain parts be inspected or replaced. Unfortunately, people usually wait for pain to occur before caring for their joints. Some damaged joints can be surgically replaced, but in this author's opinion, inspecting your posture and motion is the best solution to keep the joints you are born with working and aging well.

172|

Adaptation and the Controlling System: The Brain, Nerves and Receptors

The brain and nerves of the Control system not only control how we move, they also control our awareness of how we think we are moving, as well as the possibilities of how we can move. Like all other tissues, nerves get better at doing whatever they do. And if you never use a nerve function, you lose it. In fact, one classic Nobel Prize winning experiment showed that kittens who had an eye patch over one eye for six months permanently lost the ability to see out of that eye because crucial nerve function was lost[lxiv].

We learned earlier how patterns in the Control system, or muscle memory, can be positive (such as when we learn to type or golf and develop a "groove," or even when we learn to compensate for a limp) or negative. Negative muscle memory, called "sensory motor amnesia[lxv]," is when we literally forget how to move in some patterns of motion. People usually find the idea of amnesia to be a bit unsettling, but like a kitten blinded by never seeing, when controlling nerves are neglected we can lose function without ever knowing it's gone.

»TRY THIS: *Hand Stretch*

In the Balance chapter we learned how proprioceptors, tiny sensors in muscles and ligaments, tell the brain when they're under mechanical stress. These are not the stress sensors sending the message "it hurts" from stretching a joint by bending a normal finger backward. Rather, the proprioceptors unconsciously signal the brain to send information about how much stress there is on a joint.

In order to move, we must relax the opposing muscle when we contract a muscle. The muscle relaxes based on proprioceptive joint stress information. Since these nerves connect in the spinal cord, not the brain, this is a completely unconscious reflex over which we have no control whatsoever. So when muscles are chronically tight and never lengthen, in addition to mechanically keeping the opposing muscles long, neurologically the opposing muscles are being sent signals that make it difficult to use them. The ten-dollar name for this is Sherrington's Law of Reciprocal Inhibition, but it simply means we unconsciously relax the biceps every time we contract our triceps.

Hand Stretch demonstrates a clinical muscle therapy technique called PNF (proprioceptive neuromuscular facilitation), which uses unconscious reflexes to relax tight muscle fibers by activating others.

1. Note how far back you can bend your left wrist.

2. Take your right hand and bend it back to the beginning edge of mild discomfort for 10 seconds.

3. Now, continue holding with your right hand, but also push back with the left hand for 8 seconds.

4. Maintain pressure with the right hand, but let the left one go about half way back up to neutral.

5. Then relax the left hand and note how far back you can go.

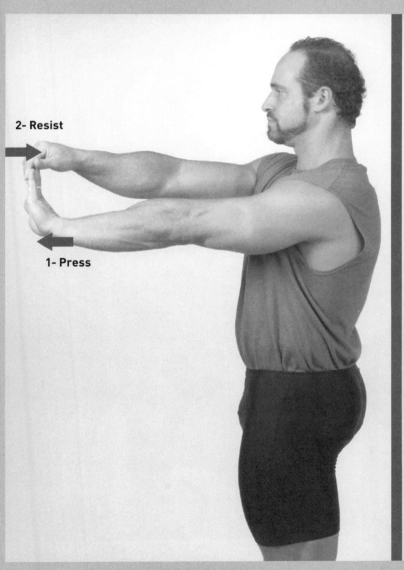

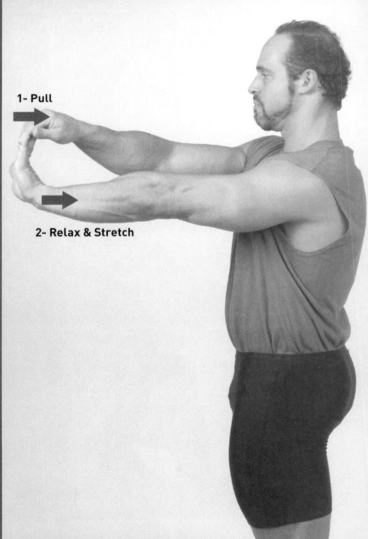

2- Resist

1- Press

1- Pull

2- Relax & Stretch

Figure 8-6 Hand stretch

174|

PNF Stretching:

Telling nerves to tell muscles to relax.

Many trainers use PNF stretching techniques to improve muscle stretches. With a partner, try this hamstring PNF stretch:

1. Lie flat on the floor with your knees straight.

2. Have a partner flex your knee upward to where you feel some gentle resistance.

3. Keeping the knee to your chest, have your partner resist as you push your foot down against their resistance for 8 seconds.

4. Then slowly release as your partner continues to gently straighten your knee until they feel slight resistance.

Most people note an increase in how high their leg comes up. (Note: Do not do this if you are experiencing acute back pain and stop at the first sign of any discomfort.)

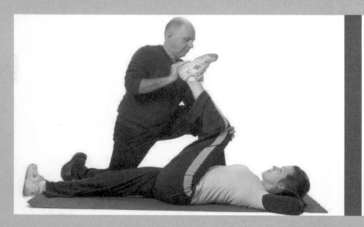
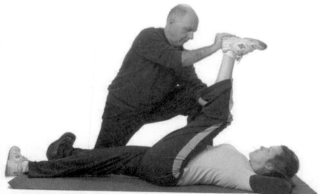

▲ **Figure 8-7** Hamstring PNF Stretch

Changes in Posture and Motion cause the Body to Change

So not only do muscles and ligaments adapt, but plasticity in brain and nerves[lxvi] cause physical changes from how they are used, stressed, and stimulated as compensation and adaptation train the Control system. "Nerves that fire together, wire together," strengthening the connection between neurons that are active at the same time. On the other hand, "Neurons that fire out of sync, lose their link," meaning that when a nerve's timing is off, function suffers[lxvii]. It's not just use it or lose it, but according to prominent neuroscientist Mark Bear, inappropriate nervous system activity is worse than no activity at all[lxviii].

Long-term ligament stress (such as when weak muscles compensate and shift stress to a joint capsule or other ligament) train proprioceptive sensors to get better at doing what they do, which is telling the brain something is amiss. Consciously the sensation may fade into the background as we perceive nothing or only low grade pain, but profound changes occur as posture adapts and changes how you stand, sit, walk, climb a flight of stairs, and move in daily life. In fact, damage to proprioceptors from old injuries not only causes weak balance, but proprioceptors sending wrong information to the brain is associated with chronic back pain[lxix].

As a result, negative and positive muscle memory reinforces the mechanical adaptations of ligaments stretching or tightening and muscles strengthening or weakening to create patterns of motion that are as powerful as they are unconscious.

So in addition to adaptation of architecture (Contracting and Connecting systems), the brain and nerves of the Control system progressively change over time as imbalanced body motion and misaligned joint stress progressively stretch some ligaments and tighten others, and overused muscles become chronically tight and underused partner muscles weaken.

Your injuries and LifeHabits create folds in your unique BodyType to literally become part of how your body moves as adaptation creates posture patterns in how we move and balance. Adaptive patterns of body motion increase body stress, breakdown, and premature aging as we get better at moving with poor posture and body motion patterns, for worse. . .

. . . *or for better*

"Use it to Keep it"

The posture principle of Adaptation is a two-edged blade. Just as posture compensation and adaptive motion prematurely ages the body, if we regularly fully move previously neglected muscles and joints, we can move well as we age.

It is important to note that with posture and body motion, we are talking about vicious spirals, not merely vicious circles. A vicious cycle is when something causes more of that something. We see vicious cycles in many aspects of life. Overweight people are more sedentary, so they eat more, exercise less, and gain more weight. Lonely people are unhappy and stay home, so they don't meet other people, and the people they meet frequently don't care to make a new friend of an unhappy person. When we speak of the Pain Cycle, we are really talking about a vicious spiral, because as posture and motion become progressively worse, increased mechanical stress on the joints creates more wear and tear, deconditioning, and progressively more breakdown, arthritis, and joint degeneration.

The vicious spiral of the Pain Cycle can be slowed, and even reversed with conscious, focused motion exercises designed to counteract the asymmetry of sitting. Along with other intelligent LifeHabits, restoring free, balanced motion reduces joint stress, relieves pain, and restores flexibility to break the Pain Cycle. The goal of training StrongPosture™ is to create a Motion Cycle and train muscles to be strong, flexible, and in control for ease of motion and vitality as you age.

176|

The Motion Cycle

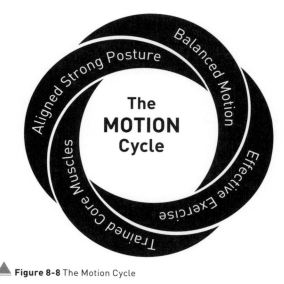

▲ **Figure 8-8** The Motion Cycle

Aligned, StrongPosture™

The Motion Cycle begins with StrongPosture™ aligned so strong core muscles smoothly guide and provide a stable platform for all the muscles in the kinetic chain. It's no coincidence that strengthening these core muscles also improves balance, since your posture is literally how you balance your body (1st Posture Principle).

There is no one "perfect" posture, just as there is no one "perfect" exercise routine. But every exercise instructor, trainer, or teacher will tell you to "watch your form. " Good form is everything, according to all fitness experts. Some may stress it more than others, but no one argues with the importance of good posture.

Theoretically, if you just did what Grandma said and "Sit up straight," then, over time, a new posture will become more of a habit. Even though it seems logical that posture should improve if we just try to sit straight, unfortunately we can't always think about our posture. Merely pulling your shoulders back to "sit up straight" doesn't work for more than thirty seconds because we have adapted to poor posture and strengthened the muscles of poor posture.

Balance exercises help combat gravity by reprogramming posture to align where you think your body and posture is in space with the reality of your posture and how your body is really moving. Challenging balance overstresses the Control system so proprioceptive and stabilizing muscles fire and seldom used muscles and nerve pathways are recruited.

When you sit on a ball, if you think you are sitting straight but in reality you are leaning to the left, you will fall to the left. But as you feel your body moving, you compensate and internal feedback helps your balance with the external reality.

Conscious focus on motion, as in WallTilts, BallTilts, yoga or Pilates, is essential to re-train posture-controlling core muscles for strong balance and strong motion. Performing StrongPosture™ exercises in front of a mirror can help keep you symmetrical and aware of body alignment. If your body does not appear aligned, consider consulting a posture professional, because strong aligned posture sets the stage for balanced, full range motion.

Balanced, Full Range Motion

Symmetrical motion within a joint's full range balances and distributes mechanical forces, so stress is distributed. The body adapts to get better at doing whatever you do, so working all of the body's joints in their full ranges, on a regular basis, can help weak muscles strengthen, tight muscles stretch, and ligaments adapt for StrongPosture™ and body motion. Therefore, ideal exercise works all the joints and all the muscles, in balance, in all possible directions.

When joint motion has been lost, professional intervention may be necessary. Chiropractic adjustments can restore long-lost mobility and deep muscle therapy such as Graston™, Rolfing, Active Release™, Trigger point, or other deep massage therapy make it possible to train muscles in their full range. However, it is then important to keep that motion with a StrongPosture™ exercise LifeHabit to work muscles and joints in the ways they do not otherwise move. Regardless of how you do it, exercises that work muscles in the positions and angles of StrongPosture™ and alignment, strengthen weak muscles, stretch tight muscles, and improve core muscle coordination so you get the most benefit out of your exercise.

Balanced, Effective Exercise

"You can't get there from here." American Folk Saying

Effective exercise means muscles fully lengthen and then fully contract. Muscle fibers contract fully or not at all, so when a joint doesn't move in a full range, exercise is less effective because the muscle fibers that should contract during an unused arc of motion are not used.

Training people to exercise with strong and stable posture and conscious, full range, normally coupled motion helps break the Pain Cycle. When people suffering with back, neck, or other muscle and joint pain learn to move in ways that reduce the stress on weak areas, and then strengthen weaknesses, mechanical stress is reduced and balance, motion, and function improves. Exercising with StrongPosture™ helps you get the most out of your exercise so you look, feel, and age well.

There is no one perfect exercise. Aerobic exercise where the whole body is moving continuously uses the large muscles and raises the heart rate, and is necessary for cardiovascular health according to the American College of Sports Medicine. Basic strength conditioning to maintain (or add) muscle mass is important, and has been shown to improve balance in older adults[lxx]. Weights or elastic bands can help strengthen muscle tissue. The important thing is to do something you enjoy so it becomes part of your life. And beginning whatever you do with StrongPosture™ helps ensure you get maximum benefits from your exercise. Conscious posture is a beginning, not an end.

It is astounding how many books on the market demonstrate exercises with poor posture awareness. Look at one of the dozens (or is it hundreds) of exercise books at your bookstore. Look at the models and observe, How is their posture? Are they symmetrical? Are their feet angled and spaced equally? Are their arms and hands facing equally on both sides?

A new patient with a back problem recently told me that she tried Pilates, but it hurt her low back and so stopped. Behaviorally, people who are hurt by exercise avoid it, further feeding the Pain Cycle.

If a body is not in balance, exercising places even greater

unbalanced stress on the muscles and joints as people use the strong muscles and avoid the weak ones. Once you have a problem you keep on moving adaptively. So in addition to being deconditioned, people who do not exercise literally cannot move normally, and move in ways which create pain, perpetuating imbalances and setting the stage for further adaptation and new injury.

I have seen people exercising in the gym using "trick," adaptive motions to unintentionally train poor posture. You might be able to lift a few more pounds by doing a bench press twisting your shoulders and jutting your head forward, but don't be surprised when you develop rotator cuff or neck problems.

Chiropractors and physical therapists, yoga instructors, and personal trainers all agree: To keep all the muscles strong, you must exercise symmetrically and with proper form.

motion , which is why many experts agree core stabilization is important to prevent low back pain.

But it's not just about pain. Strong stabilization is important in everything we do, from the athlete pursuing physical excellence to the parent lifting a child. When we learned One-Leg Balance and the Stability Challenge we saw how contracting the core muscles in a pelvic tilt helped to stabilize balance and strengthen posture.

In structure as well as in function, the hand bone really is connected to the arm bone, the arm bone is connected to the chest bone, and so on.

Trained Core Muscles

Imagine This:

Lift a 10' long, 50 pound pipe and carry it across the street.
Now imagine the pipe turning to flexible rubber.
Which pipe would be easier to carry?

It's easier to lift a rigid object that doesn't flop around and can be balanced well. We saw in the Broom Balance demo how posture is strong when you balance the head over the torso, the torso over the pelvis, and the pelvis over the legs. As with a floppy pipe, when the core of the body is floppy, it is more difficult to balance.

Strong core muscles create a strong and stable mechanical connection between the torso and the pelvis and are essential for effective body balance.

Research shows people with low back pain and weak posture[lxxi] do not properly stabilize the low back in daily

»TRY THIS: *Arm Lift Demo*

The arm lift demonstration shows how deep low back muscles must contract in order for you to lift your arm.

Sit up straight.

Touch your low back with your right hand, just at the waistline.

Let the tips of your fingers touch the edge or the bumps in the middle of your spine (these are the spinous process of the spinal vertebrae, bones which chiropractors look at a lot).

Now, slowly lift your left hand and feel for muscle contraction in your low back.

Can you lift your arm without tightening your low back muscles?

The contraction in the low back you are feeling is the multifidus (a deep core muscle) working to stabilize the torso on the pelvis. Everything in the kinetic chain is connected, so when you lift your arm, to hold it up you must stabilize your shoulders on your torso, and your torso on your pelvis. StrongPosture™ and motion means a strong core smoothly controlling the links of the kinetic chain. It isn't surprising that you can identify people with a history of low back pain even when they are not currently in pain by observing if multifidus contraction is delayed when they lift their arm[lxxii].

▼ **Figure 8-9** Arm lift demo

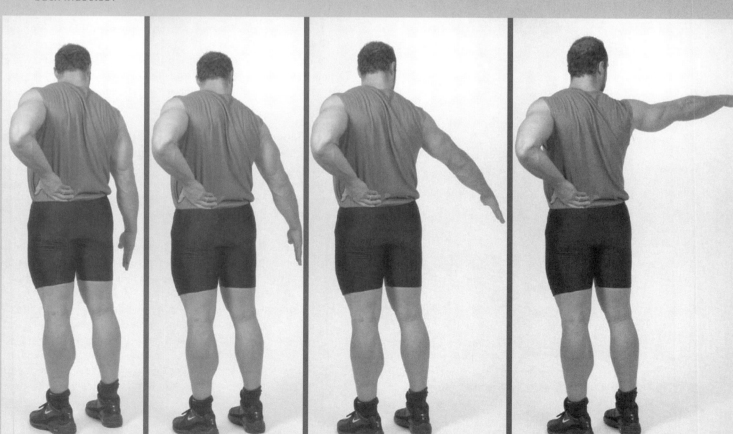

180|

Cycles can be vicious or virtuous. Pain cycles result in progressive loss of function. But focused motion exercises train strong core muscles, creating a motion cycle of strong balance, StrongPosture™, and strong core muscles to slow and even reverse the Pain Cycle. Unlocking motion and reducing tension and spasm with StrongPosture™ not only relieves pain and aligns the joints to work as they are designed to, but helps us move, balance, and even age more effectively.

It only takes a few minutes a day to create an awareness of how we move our body and wake up unused muscles.

Since posture is how you balance your body, someone who can balance well usually has better posture than someone with poor balance.

The athlete in training, the computer worker, the mom, and the construction worker can all experience dramatic changes and benefit from well-balanced, stable posture, which in turn promotes full, balanced motion.

The flip side of "Use it or lose it" is "Use it to keep it"

If we don't know there is a problem, we will never look for a solution. When standing balance is weak, motion adapts to compensate and maintain balance. Someone unaware of their adaptive posture and "trick" motions thinks they're moving naturally, but when exercising they work and strengthen an adaptive motion.

Strengthening the core muscles with these StrongPosture™ Exercises should also be part of your daily exercise because motion begins with the core. Our bodies learn what we teach them and motion follows the path of least resistance, so imbalances from injury or bad LifeHabits cause adaptive patterns that avoid the weaker core muscles.

Yoga, Pilates, Alexander Technique, and other disciplines also teach core muscle, controlled motion exercises to create posture awareness and help people "stand taller." However, even experienced practitioners of these disciplines report improved alignment and control with wall and ball StrongPosture™ exercises. All bodies are different and there is no one right exercise for all bodies and all minds. I encourage you to personally try different types and styles of exercise to find what works for you. Many who try yoga, Pilates,

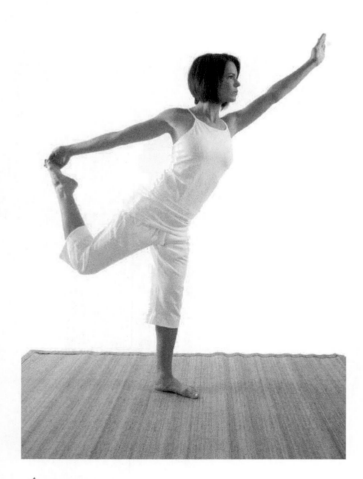

▲ **Figure 8-10** Yoga is known for building posture awareness

|181

or something else they "never thought they would like" find it is just what they have always been looking for. Then, if you like, go on to learn more with personalized attention from the appropriate instructor, coach, teacher, or trainer.

But there is more to this book than just StrongPosture™ Exercise. . . it's about becoming conscious of how you use and move your body in all parts of life, from lifting to sitting, from stretching to relaxing. Posture Angels are the culmination of the Wall Strong Alignment exercises for strong alignment, a one-minute exercise you can do anytime to align your perception of standing straight with the reality of a straight wall.

You are doing what you are doing, not what you think you are doing

Posture consciousness complements ANY exercise program. To get the most out of any exercise, you must do it correctly, so adding posture training to your daily exercise or routine aligns where you think your body and posture are in space with the reality of your posture and how your body is really moving.

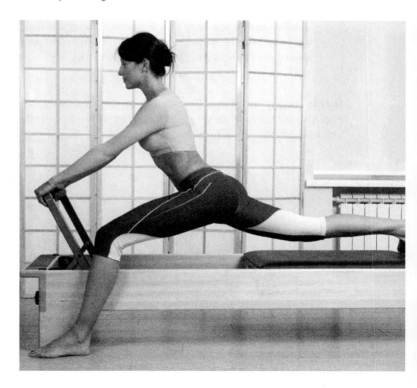

Figure 8-11 Pilates is known for building core strength ▶

StrongPosture™ Alignment:
Posture Angels

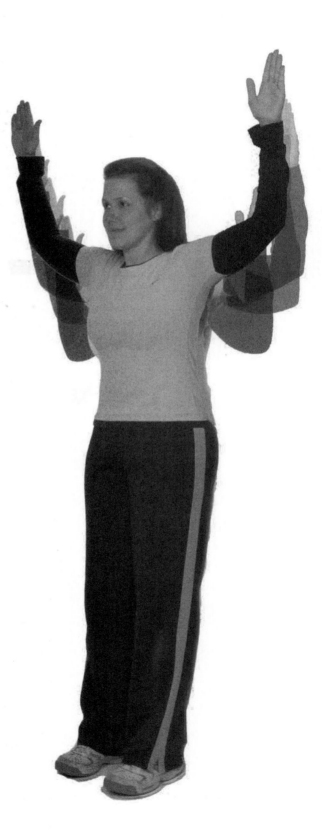

Purpose: Shoulder blade retraction, shoulder and arm motion coordinated with core motion.

Posture Angels integrate control of all four posture zones: head, torso, pelvis, and lower extremities. Since the body moves in whole motions, to change your motion programs you must consciously move in a new pattern of motion. Posture Angels effectively "wake up" and work the core muscles in a biomechanically intelligent pattern, with coordinated shoulder girdle and pelvic motion along with coordinating breathing and head and spinal stabilization.

> Many of my chiropractic patients also use Posture Angels as their barometer for when they need to be adjusted. When I walk into a room to adjust these wellness patients they do a Posture Angel to find locks in their kinetic chain, deep spasm, and other motion problems. After I adust them, they go back to the wall to re-check their Posture Angel to see if they feel as good as they know they can. Regular StrongPosture™ exercise really does make a difference in your awareness of how your body is moving, so when it stiffens up you can do something about it.

Goal: Doing an ArmsUP pelvic tilt while adding the coordinated vertical raising and lowering of the forearms, and keeping the shoulders level and stable.

Figure 8-12 Posture Angel ▶

1. Aware Posture:

Leaning against a wall- Are the:

> Feet hip distance apart, a foot from the wall?

>> Feet parallel, with the heels and toes equidistant and toes pointing straight forward?

> Buttocks pressed against the wall?

> Knees straight and strong, not bent or hyper-extended?

> Arms against the wall, equally spaced from the body?

> Palms facing forward?

> Head level but pressed to wall as far as possible, with eyes facing forward?

2. Conscious Motion:

> Begin by doing a WallTilt,
>> Arch and breathe IN
>>> Then tuck in a WallTilt as you breathe out

> Then an ArmsUp WallTilt, and
>> Breathe IN, arch and lift arms into ArmsUp
>>> Breathe out and tuck,

> Then progress into a PostureAngel.
>> Arch your pelvis, breathe IN and

> Raise your hands toward the ceiling
>> Keep:
>> - Elbows against wall
>> - Forearms perpendicular to the floor
>> - Wrists and forearms aligned

Tuck your pelvis, breathe out and
> Pull arms down. Keep forearms perpendicular to the floor

Coordinate pelvic arching and breathing with controlled arm motion for 5 slow breaths.

TIPS:

Remember: The goal is to be conscious of every degree of motion as you PRESS the tuck, and only gently EXPLORE the arch.

Breathe in and Arch your pelvis gently,

And reach your arms up as your buttocks slide toward the ceiling.

Breathe out and Tuck your pelvis

And gently pull your arms down, keeping your wrists straight, fingers pointing to the ceiling.

Push your tailbone toward the floor and your big toe into the ground.

Arch and gently breathe in

Keep your elbows pressed against the wall as you slowly reach for the ceiling.

Tuck your pelvis, press firmly, and fully exhale

And pull your arms toward the floor.

Pull your shoulder blades together.

Tilt your pubic bone up, and in, toward your belly button.

Slowly and gently explore the arch with your breath

Keep your head level and forearms parallel.

Tuck firmly and exhale

With flowing motion, keep your head level and facing forward, press your head into the wall.

Flatten your back so your belly button pushes back to the wall.

Arch and breathe in

With flowing motion, reach your hands for the sky, pressing

the pinky to the wall.

Roll your thighs gently together.

Exhale fully and tuck

Keep your pinky to the wall as your elbows come down, forearms parallel, shoulder blades toward one another.

Arch and breathe in as your buttocks gently slide up toward the ceiling

Keep your head stable and level as your hands slide up.

Tuck and exhale fully

Press your head and your hands to the wall as your elbows point to the floor. Keep your wrists perfectly straight.

CUEING TIPS

Posture Angels, along with all other StrongPosture™ Exercises, should be performed slowly and timed by your breathing. When you breathe and move slowly you recruit and activate unused muscle fibers from neglected parts of a joint's arc of motion. Slow, breath-controlled motion creates posture consciousness from the bottom to the top of the kinetic chain.

When you tuck, breathe out and:

■ pull your belly in,

■ roll your thighs together,

■ press your big toe into the floor,

■ rotate the bottom of your spine (tailbone) under your body (imagine a puppy putting his tail between his legs).

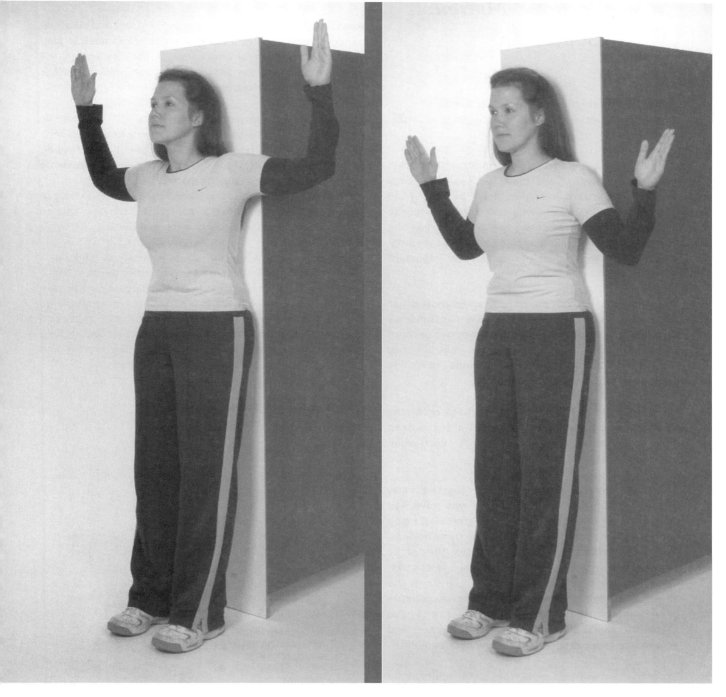

 Figure 8-13a Posture Angel with weak neck stabilization -note looking up posture

Figure 8-13b Posture Angel with weak shoulder stabilization -note arms winging out

StrongPosture™ Motion:
Superman

Purpose: Promote coupled spinal motion
Strengthen core deep spinal stabilization muscles

Just as the Posture Angel focuses you on StrongPosture™ alignment on the wall, Superman focuses your core muscles and spine toward StrongPosture™ by moving and balancing on the ball. Your twenty-four spinal vertebrae should all be able to move, and the Superman progressions are fantastic for waking up and working the deepest spinal muscles (called the multifidus) as well as other important back muscles such as erector spinae.

The unique thing about multifidus versus most other spinal muscles is that multifidus are one-joint muscles while the other spinal muscles go across two or more joints. When the one-joint muscles contract they "lock" two vertebrae together and provide the rigidity necessary for us to stabilize our body.

MRIs of people with a history of low back problems show there is an actual loss of mass of these deep muscles on the side of low back pain. . . even when someone is not in pain[lxxiii, lxxiv]!

Also, EMGs measuring the electrical muscle activity of these muscles show that people who have had back pain move their body with less symmetry, using patterns of motion that are different from normal. As they go through their daily activities, they place dramatically greater bio-mechanical stress on the spine, discs, and other joints. . . . even in the absence of any symptoms[lxxv, lxxvi]. However, patients performing focused StrongPosture™ exercises have shown increased size of these deep stabilizers and experience fewer recurrences of low back pain[lxxvii].

So, in order to move well you must train all the joints of the body to move fully. We coordinate the motion of opposing muscles to keep ourselves stable as we move, so it is not surprising that spinal stress and injury often result from a failure of coordination rather than from actual weakness[lxxviii]. Back extensors must contract and lengthen as torso flexors contract and shorten to keep a back strong. Weakness and loss of endurance of back extensors not only correlate with low back pain, but can predict whether someone will suffer low back problems in the future[lxxix, lxxx].

The goal of the Superman StrongPosture™ exercise is controlled full extension of the torso from a flexed position.
First, the BallHug helps relieve pain by de-stressing the spinal joints, fully opening the joints and allowing spinal muscles to lengthen.
Then, Superman is a slow controlled spinal extension with focus on smooth control to activate unused muscle fibers, especially in the multifidus.

If someone has a "jerky" motion when extending in Superman they are "skipping a level" either because there is no motion possible at that level of the spine, or because they have learned to move in a pattern avoiding motion in part of the spine. Slow, controlled Superman extension exercises wake up vital, deep stabilizing muscles to help prevent injury and back pain by retraining motion and breaking adaptive, or "trick," motion patterns.

Goal: Spinal Extension (active)

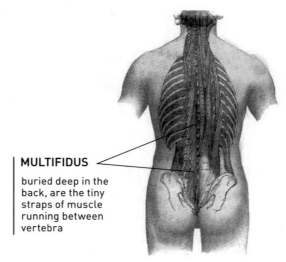

MULTIFIDUS

buried deep in the back, are the tiny straps of muscle running between vertebra

 Figure 8-14 Multifidus muscles lose strength and atrophy, resulting in weak posture and back pain.

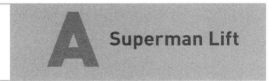

Superman Lift

MOTION: From BallHug, stabilize the body from the bottom up:

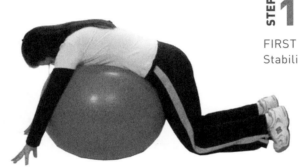

STEP 1

FIRST
Stabilize your feet, hip distance apart and parallel
Tip: Try propping your feet against a wall
for more stability.

◀ **Figure 8-15** Superman Start position

STEP 2

Lock knees

▼ **Figure 8-16** Superman Knee Lock

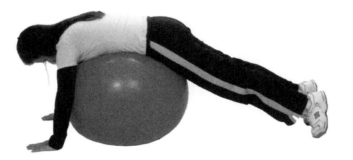

STEP 3

Tuck pelvis
Tucking pelvis protects from overextending low
back, which can cause or aggravate a problem
Retract neck
Raise arms in front of you, palms facing one another,
keeping the arms next to the ears

▼ **Figure 8-17** Superman StrongPosture™

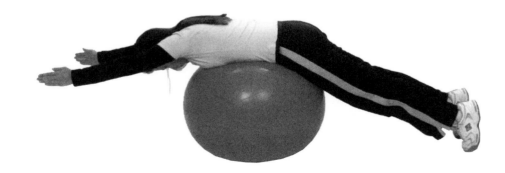

B Superman Flow

THEN
> Keeping the body in a straight line
>> knees locked, pelvis tucked, neck retracted,
>> and arms next to ears
> Lift the body up with control keeping everything in line
>> DON'T LOOK UP -Lock the arms next to your ears
> Reach up and out like Superman.

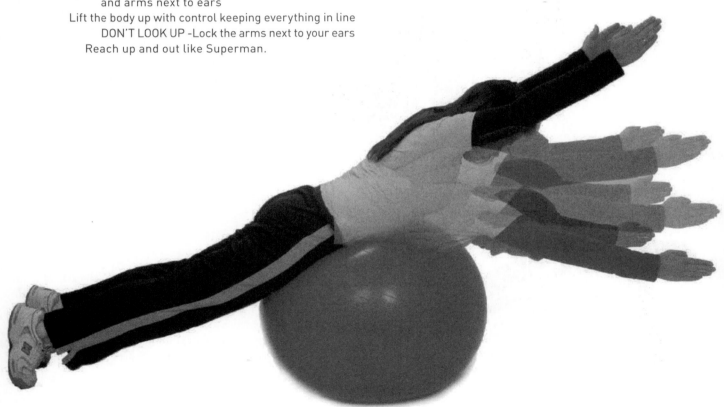

▲ **Figure 8-18** Up, up, and away!

C Superman Down

Lift your body with smooth motion as you breathe in
Lower your body with control.
Keep your knees locked, pelvis tucked, and arms
next to your ears as you lower your torso with
StrongPosture™

1

Lower your body as you breathe out.
Let your breath control and guide your motion.

▼ **Figure 8-19** Superman Down- Lower Torso,
then lose tuck

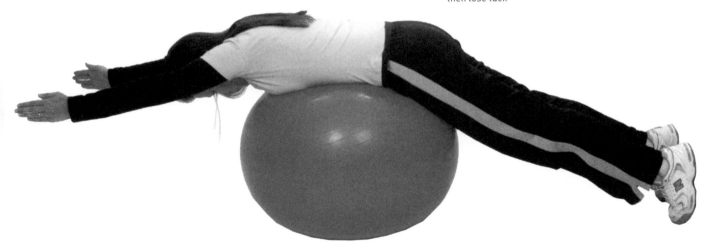

2

Repeat with slow, conscious control for 5 slow breaths
BREATHING:
Since the ball is pressing on your stomach, breathing
is reversed (breathe in on exertion), so
    Breathe IN as you go up
    Breathe OUT as you go down.

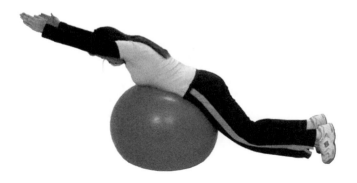

◀ **Figure 8-20** Then allow knees to bend

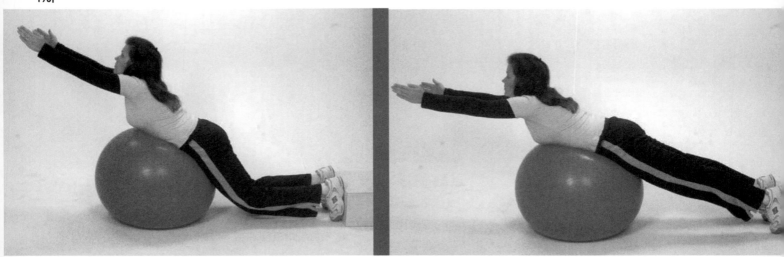

▲ **Figure 8-21** Incorrect Superman

PEELBACKS:

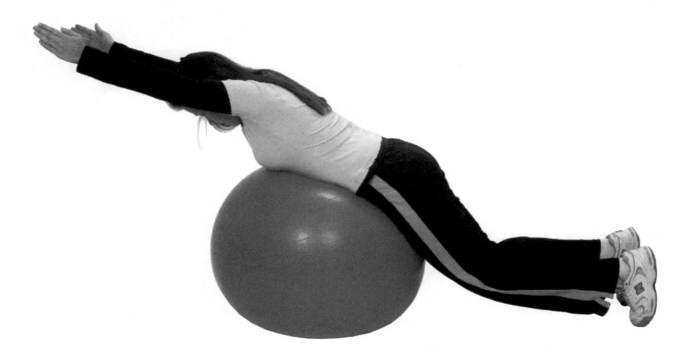

▲ **Figure 8-22** Superman Peelback

PROGRESSIONS:

It is far better to do any exercise with good form than to strain and use poor form. Since we are putting the spine into an extended position, Superman progressions *especially* should only be attempted if you can do basic Superman with good form and control. Once you learn strong full body core stabilization with a Posture Angel, you or a Certified Posture Exercise Professional (CPEP) may decide to emphasize, deemphasize, or omit exercises based on your body type and history. Listen to your body. Hippocrates, the father of healing, advised physicians to "Above all, do no harm," and this holds for those of us who want to care for our own bodies.

Hold your body up in a Superman for up to 3 breaths. Try Superman holding your feet together.

Rolling forward on the ball lets us add other exercises to a daily StrongPosture™ exercise progression. Here are some ideas to try:

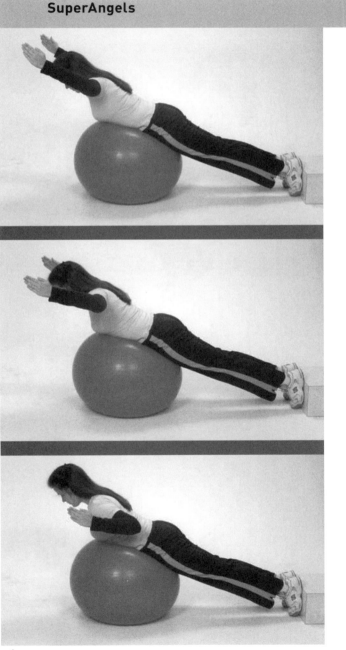

SuperAngels

▲ **Figure 8-24** SuperAngels

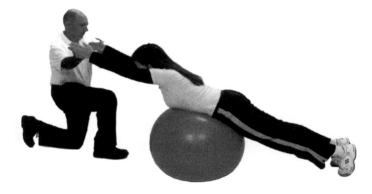

▲ **Figure 8-23** Assisted Superman

192|

Leg Lifts

Keep your pelvis tucked and do not over-arch the low back

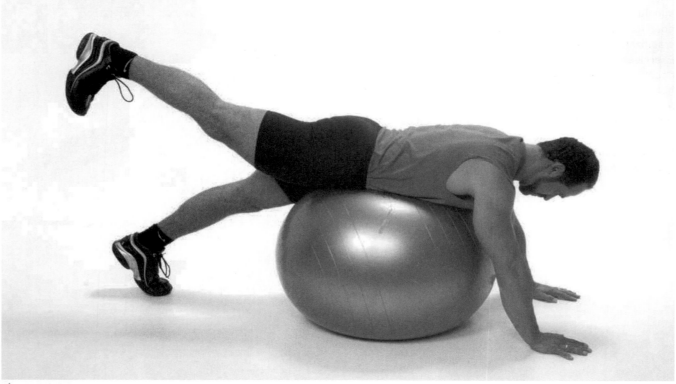

▲ **Figure 8-25** Leg Lifts

Cross Crawl

Great for whole body stability

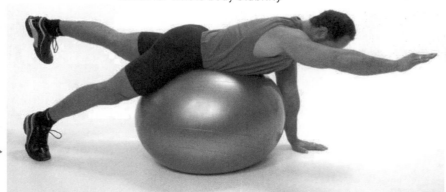

Figure 8-26 Cross Crawl ▶

Rollouts

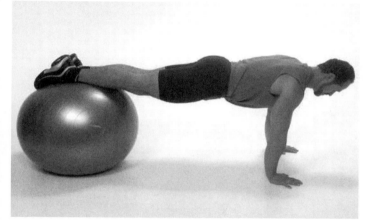

Figure 8-27 Rollouts ▲

Ball PushUp

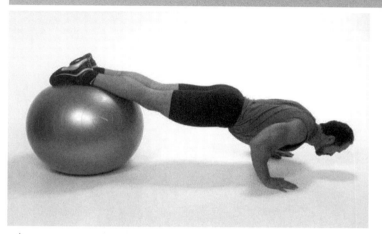

▲ **Figure 8-28** Ball PushUp

RollOut AbCrunch

▼ **Figure 8-29** RollOut AbCrunch

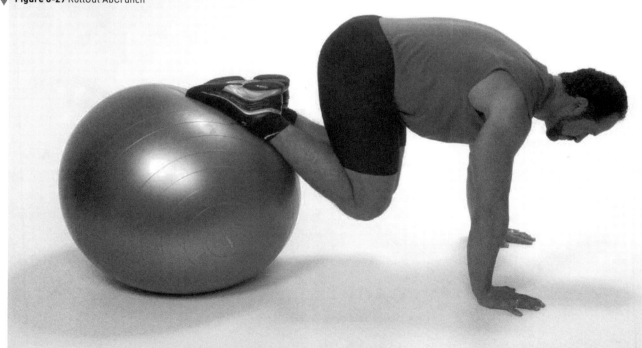

Ball Down Dog

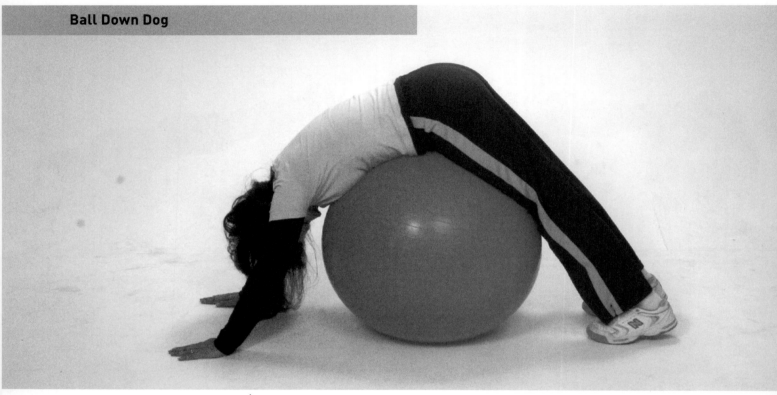

▲ **Figure 8-30** Ball DownDog

Renee's Challenge

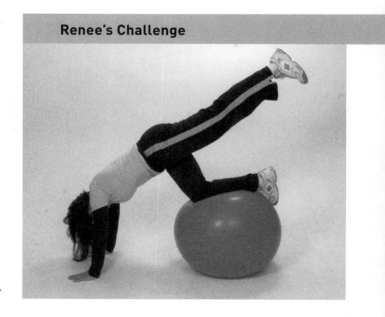

Figure 8-31 Renee´s Challenge ▶

StrongPosture™
7 Week Program-

B
A
M

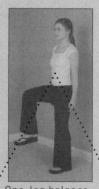

One-leg balance
(**The Stork**)-p.19

Strong Balance

BALANCE **3** times a day

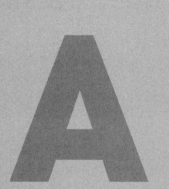

WallTilt -p66

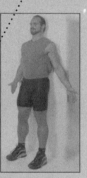

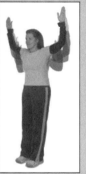

Posture Angels -p.182

Strong Alignment

ALIGNMENT **2** times a day

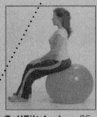

BallTilt Arch -p.75

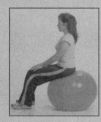

BallTilt Tuck -p.75

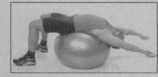

BallStretch -p.101

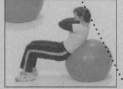

AbFocus -p.131

MOTION **1** once a day

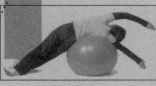

SideStretch -p.103

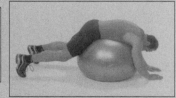

BallHug -p.159

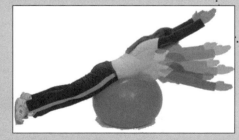

Superman -p.187

Strong Motion

196|

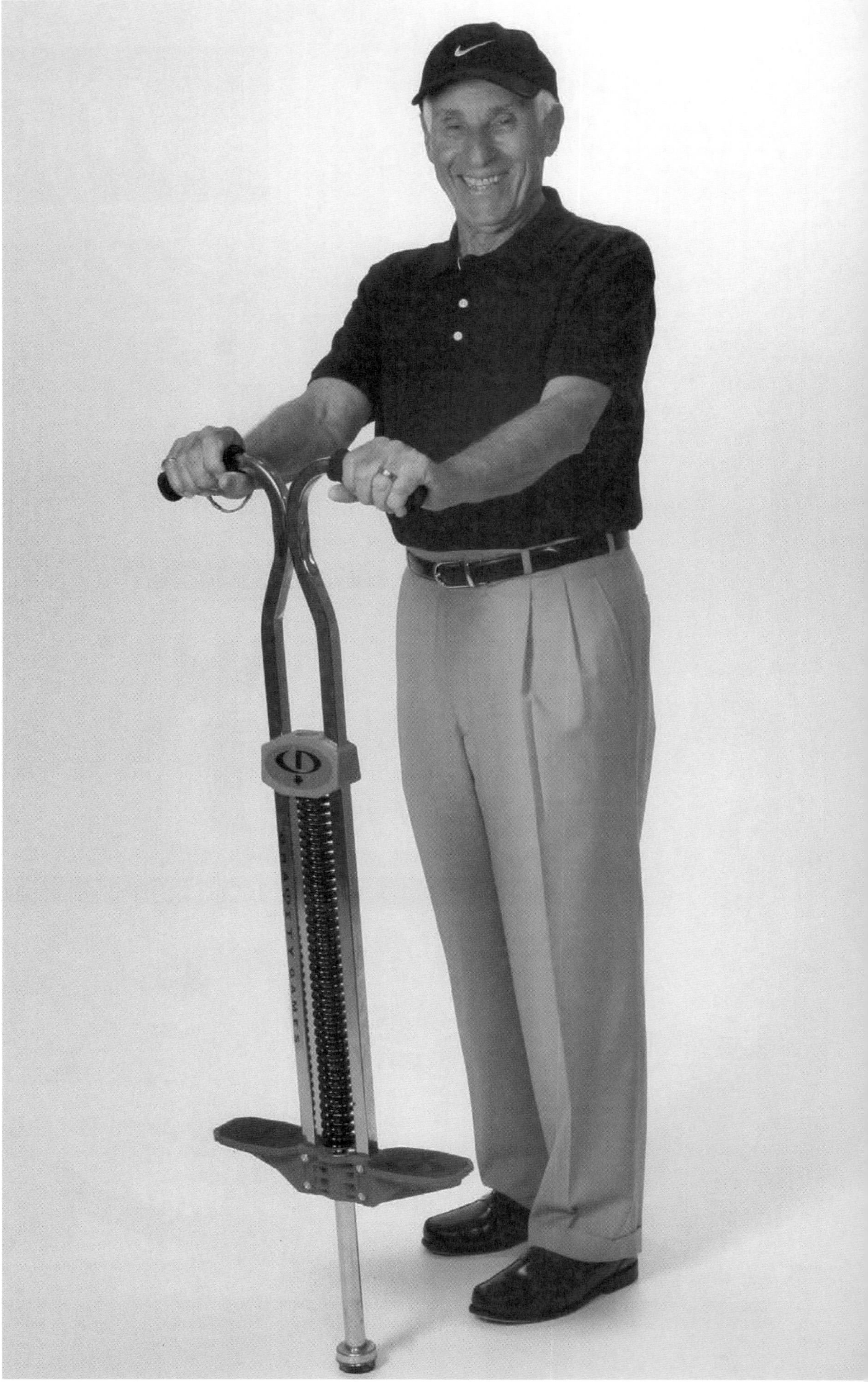

9 StrongPosture™
A LifeHabit for Intelligent Aging

> *"Mens sana in corpore sano"*
> *(A healthy mind in a healthy body)*
> Juvenal, Roman author (55 AD - 127 AD)

Figure 9-1 Stand Taller and Live Longer

Aging Boomers in the 21st Century

The first step in solving a problem is defining it. The second is executing a solution.

This book began by defining the problem of 21st century habits prematurely aging our bodies, and then presented a program for daily StrongPosture™ Exercises that can not only prevent many of the consequences of our sitting LifeHabits, but also actually help people live healthier and, yes, even longer.

Lifespan is how long you live. Healthspan is how long you live well. People have always wanted to live many years, and no one wants to feel sick and unable to care for themselves or enjoy life. However, we live in a unique time, and for the next few decades, living well as well as living longer will be increasingly important for a unique reason: the impending biological revolution.

198| Just as the machine age morphed into the computer age, we live at the dawn of the biological age. The first decade or so of the 21st century will be recorded by history as the beginning of a biological revolution, which will rival (and possibly surpass) the electronics revolution of the past half century.

From decoding the human genome to customized treatments based on your genotype, biology today is poised to be this century's revolution. The first decade of the 21st century is already showing astounding advances making it a safe bet that if you can live, and keep your body working well for another twenty or thirty years, technologies will become available to keep you active and healthy for far longer than your grandfather lived with genetics similar to yours.

> **My prediction:** Just as 1990's consumers held off buying a new computer, waiting for a faster one next year, over the next 2 decades aging boomers will become fanatically health conscious, desperate to keep healthy long enough to benefit from the next year's new technology.

So what can we do today to live long enough, and stay healthy enough, to enjoy these benefits? Unfortunately, experts don't agree on everything. Some promote the value of screening tests for everything and annual checkups, while others argue over whether early detection means better results or merely knowing about something longer. Others receive regular chiropractic adjustments, massage, and take different nutritional supplements. Many (including myself) try to avail themselves of the best of both traditional and alternative therapies.

Products tout health and long life, as apparent in any supermarket or health food store. However, even for those with research behind the claims, their relative effectiveness may be marginal (Remember the diet fad of drinking 8 glasses of ice cold water a day on the true theory that calories are heat? The premise was that warming the water to body temperature required 120 calories, so you would lose an extra pound a month. Sounds good, until you realize heat is measured in calories, and food is measured in kilocalories, or 1000 heat calories, so instead of a pound a month it comes out to a pound every 80 years).

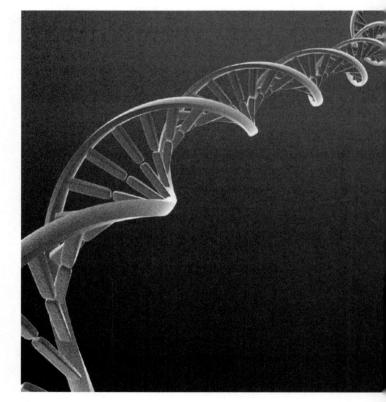

▲ **Figure 9-2** HealthSpan is determined by your DNA and your Daily LifeHabits

7 LifeHabits for a Long HealthSpan

There are LifeHabits that almost all experts agree are effective and vitally important to living healthy as long as you can. You already know about them from numerous books and articles (as well from most of our mothers). However, they bear repeating:

1 ■ Don't smoke or use tobacco
2 ■ Eat well and maintain a healthy weight
    i. Minimize anything white (sugar, salt, flour)
    ii. Fresh is best, frying is bad
    iii. Eat more fruits and vegetables
    iv. Eat balanced meals with more good and less bad fats (more turkey, less beef)
    v. Strongly avoid high fructose corn syrup.
        1. Also known as HFCS, this form of sugar was introduced in the 1980s and has been labeled as a culprit in adding to America's expanding waistline because of its quick conversion into fat.
3 ■ Be happy in your personal and professional life
4 ■ If you drink alcohol, use moderation
5 ■ Avoid drugs and consult your doctor about minimizing your dependence on medication
6 ■ Get adjusted regularly
    i. Many older and active patients tell me one of their secrets for staying active is getting adjusted once a month.
7 ■ EXERCISE

Probably the most agreed upon LifeHabit for a long HealthSpan is **EXERCISE**. If the health benefits of exercise could be put in a pill, it would be the best selling pill on the market. Research shows that the relative health benefits of regular, consistent exercise dwarfs the benefit of other (good) LifeHabits such as a low fat diet, taking herbs, antioxidants, or other remedies to improve health. Research studies show exercise prevents joint problems, and doesn't cause wear-and-tear arthritis. Consider:

■ Regular exercise into older age...can slow age-related changes in heart rate, aerobic capacity and muscle mass. *Wall Street Journal October 2007*

■ Numerous studies show that greater physical activity is associated with decreased risk of cardiovascular disease, hypertension, diabetes and obesity. 2007 recommendations from the American Heart Association and American College of Sports Medine.

■ Lack of regular exercise can be considered a "risk factor" for the development of problems in the muscles and joints[lxxxi].

■ A 20-year Stanford University study of middle-age runners showed no more arthritis than in the non-runners, and the runners actually had a lower risk of musculo-skeletal conditions and pain[lxxxii].

■ A 25-year Cooper Institute study found no link between running and hip or knee arthritis. Runners, even long-time, heavy-mileage runners, were less likely to suffer severe hip or knee pain, or to require surgery for arthritis. After comparing 504 college runners with 287 college swimmers, the conventional training wisdom that swimming is less likely to cause arthritis than running was found to be untrue[lxxxiii].

The only way to change something is to do something different. We can remain unconscious of posture and accept the posture degeneration, low-grade pain, and overall aging before our time as the consequence, or we can choose to change how we move our body, and reap the benefit of wellbeing and the vitality of positive body changes.

2001

Conscious Motion to Shape Posture and Other Unconscious Habits

"Habits are what you do."
Stephen Covey, 7 Habits of Highly Effective People

Your body is shaped by two things: your genetics and your experiences, including injuries and habits. Your genetics, like it or not, you cannot change. Your habits, like it or not, you can choose. Most people have plenty of room for improvement in their health and exercise habits. And choices can be made, while consequences are only accepted.

Much as we might like to deny the changes of age, as well as possibly years of abuse, they are real. Gravity constantly pulls us down. Especially when posture is unbalanced, we must work harder to resist gravity and keep from falling down. And once a body has become out of shape, or deconditioned, it moves differently. If there is a protruding abdomen with a compensating forward head carriage, your body motion will change over the years to compensate. Working out a twenty-year-old body is like writing on a clean slate. Working out a forty (or sixty)–year-old body is another matter. Choosing to exercise is usually good, but choosing to exercise intelligently is better, which is why it makes sense to begin every exercise workout, as well as every day, by doing your posture exercises.

Healthy Habits and HabitKeys

"We are what we repeatedly do. Excellence, therefore, is not an act but a habit." Aristotle

Creating a Posture Exercises LifeHabit not only helps to keep a body moving well, but it also serves as an "early warning" system when a body begins to "stiffen up." Daily StrongPosture™ exercise keeps you posture-conscious and aware of how your body is moving. If and when pain or the long-term adaptive changes of poor posture cause restricted motion for more than a few days, don't give in to "old and stiff"–see a professional. When a joint cannot move full range, it cannot nourish itself and breakdown begins. Chiropractic adjustments can unlock and open locked joints, especially in the spine, not only to restore lost motion and relieve pain, but to help exercise to be effective. Massage therapy can unlock and free motion by stretching tight areas to break up muscle spasms, adhesions, and fibrotic soft tissue injuries. And if you need help doing posture exercises, a Certified StrongPosture™ exerciseProfessional (CPEP) (or clinically trained physical therapist, personal trainer, Pilates instructor, or yoga instructor) can help improve your form.

Sometimes people have a hard time getting into the groove of doing their posture exercises consistently. Making StrongPosture™ exercise a priority is vital to successfully create a new habit, and one way of creating a StrongPosture™ exercise habit is by utilizing HabitKeys.

HabitKeys are an activity, a time, or anything else in a daily routine, to which you can consciously tie, or "key," a new habit. If you do StrongPosture™ exercise when you "get a chance," my experience is that when you feel better, there is little chance you are going to do them. So, whether it is before lunch, after breakfast, when you let the dog out..WHENEVER, the key is to build a habit of fully moving joints and muscles with control, the same time and at the same point in your daily routine. Once a habit is created, it is (relatively) easy to maintain. Create a morning and afternoon HabitKey and commit to a good time and place in your daily schedule for your posture exercises.

StrongPosture™ LifeHabits & Activities of Daily Living

Bio-mechanical ideas to keep a body moving, feeling, and staying well

Strengthening posture means adding Posture Consciousness and exercise to your daily life. StrongPosture™ exercise on the wall gives you feedback about the alignment of the body so your daily habits are keeping your head, torso, pelvis, and legs straight. In addition, one-leg balance and ball exercises align your balance with reality for Strong Balance.

Since we all have posture compensations and adaptations, doing posture exercises with a mirror improves your posture and motion consciousness. Consider placing a mirror near where you eat (and work) so that if you look, you can see your posture from the side. Being aware of your posture, and seeing how others see you, is a powerful stimulus to strengthening your posture. Also, if you have a personal trainer or workout partner, have them check you for good form and StrongPosture™ . Professional or amateur, someone else can point out subtle differences in form to help you create the awareness necessary for postural change.

For most of your life you don't think about your posture—however, just as daily posture exercises can retrain posture, becoming aware of how you use your body during daily life trains your body to move more effectively. From motion and balance to patterns, compensation and ultimately the two-edged blade of adaptation, the bio-mechanics of the Posture Principles dictate that to change posture we must be aware of how we move our body. However, we can't walk around thinking about the position, alignment, and motion of the head and torso, shoulder girdle, ribcage, torso, and pelvis, and our breathing all day. We have to choose to program ourselves by creating a habit.

Following are common activities we all do, and some specific ideas on how to move with StrongPosture, balance, and motion. Tuck your pelvis, retract and align your head, pull your shoulders down and back, and breathe with your belly. In other words, what your mother always told you.

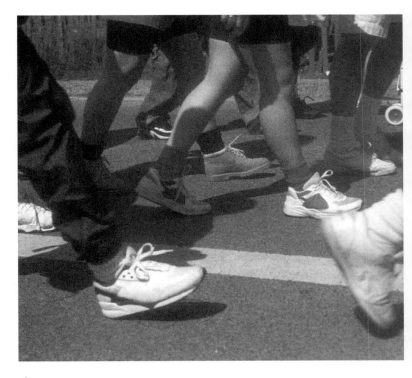

▲ **Figure 9-3** Walking is the perfect exercise

The Best Exercise LifeHabit: Walking

"What's the best exercise?" and "What's is the right amount of which kind of exercise?" are what I call "cheesecake recipe" questions. I love cheesecake (and accept it is in no way healthy), have tried hundreds of different kinds and recipes, and like some better than others, but at the end of the day picking the best one is a matter of taste. Experts argue about how long to exercise for maximum wellness benefit, but all agree it's important. Most advise exercising at least three times a week for thirty minutes, but five times a week is likely significantly better. On the other hand, if you spend three hours a day, every day, in the gym, research doesn't show it will help you live significantly longer than someone exercising consistently but more moderately[lxxxiv, lxxxv].

Walking is the perfect exercise. If you are looking for something easy to do, a brisk walk burns nearly as many calories as running the equivalent distance, with far less risk of injury. And walking with conscious StrongPosture™ helps to train a new habit and motion.

Walking Suggestions:

Necessary: Good Shoes

A good idea: Custom orthotic shoe inserts, or even over-the-counter shoe inserts. Cushioning is nice, but support is far more important. Look at a pair of your old shoes- if wear is uneven, with excessive wear on the back outside edges (indicating pronation), you are standing and walking on a lopsided platform. See a chiropractor, podiatrist, or other professional if there is pain or if off-the-shelf foot inserts are not helpful after a short trial.

»TRY THIS: *StrongWalking*

Before walking, do five Posture Angels, focusing on breathing through your nose.
Then keep your pelvis slightly tucked as you walk, and focus on strong belly breathing.

As you walk, Visualize This:
■ A helium balloon attached to the top of your head lifting you up.
■ Two helium balloons attached to your chest lifting you up.

Occasionally focus on:
■ Your big toe pushing off
■ Your heel striking the ground
■ Your sit bone going forward with your heel
■ Your right hip and left shoulder coming forward together (and then left hip and right shoulder)
■ Your neck being retracted
■ Your shoulder blades pulling together

Also, when you are ready:
■ Lift your arms into Arms UP and take 5 steps
■ Move your arms up and down in 5 "Walking Angels"

Being Smart on Your Feet: StrongStanding

People who stand at work (such as machine operators), or at home (think cooking or washing the dishes) are constantly using muscles to maintain balance. Just as walking is easier than standing because we change legs, you can balance biomechanical stress by alternating standing on one leg and then shifting to the other.

If you have to stand in one place for long periods of time during your day, create a HabitKey so you do a pelvic tilt three or four times an hour (although also finding a wall to practice WallTilts is a great idea during a break)

Also,
- Balance on one leg for three breaths
- Tuck your pelvis
- Place a box or a low shelf where you can put a foot up to switch off the postural stress.
    - When you switch legs, do a standing pelvic tilt
- **Play with your balance:** Try to put your shoes, or even your socks, on while standing up

Do Pelvic Tilts and One-Leg Balance regularly during the day—

when you brush your teeth, talk on the phone, whenever!

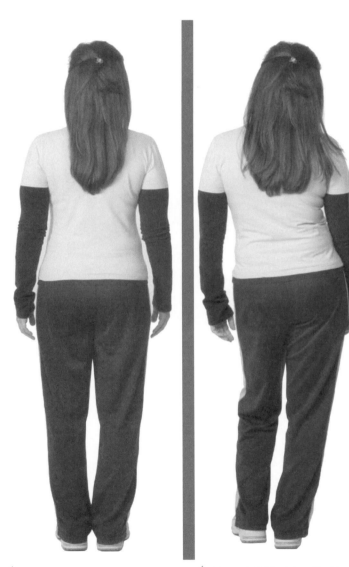

▲ **Figure 9-4a** Strong Standing Posture ▲ **Figure 9-4b** Weak Standing Posture

204|

The Ups and Downs of Stairs

When you walk up a flight of stairs notice: Does your head poke forward and your chest lean forward of your hips to balance your body as you climb stairs? If so, you must be moving your pelvis backward as well to balance, a very common pattern for people with folded and forward body motion patterns.

The solution: Hold your pelvis in a tuck as you push your chest up while climbing stairs. This forces you to hold your shoulders back and over your hips.

Wear a tie or pendant as you go up a flight of stairs. Use StrongPosture™ to be aware of your torso alignment by focusing on keeping your tie or pendant touching your body.

Or, hold an imaginary plumb line (or make a real one from a string and a pen against your chin, and go up the stairs keeping the pen against your body.

This forces you to keep your body erect, and to train your muscles to work your body in a more bio-mechanically effective pattern.

"It's amazing how conscious posture makes me feel like I am exercising every time I carry the baby upstairs." A patient

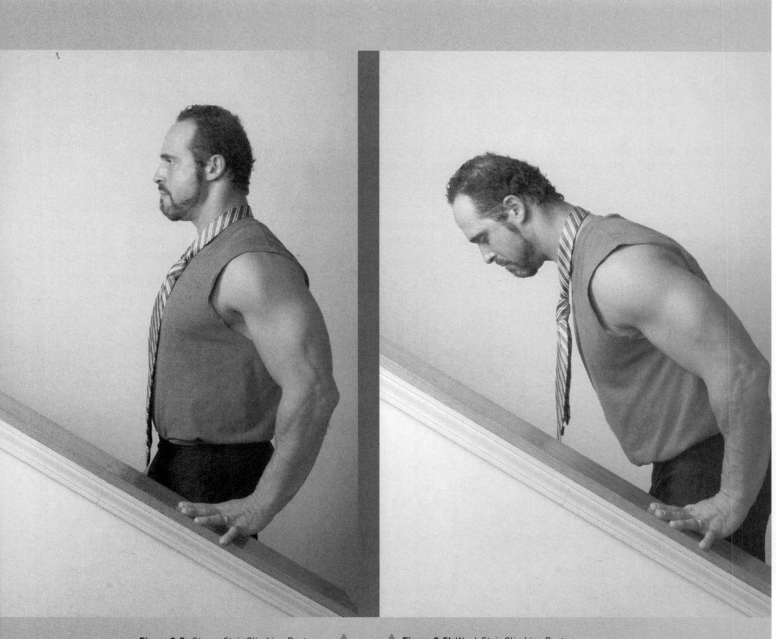

Figure 9-5a Strong Stair Climbing Posture **Figure 9-5b** Weak Stair Climbing Posture

206|

Strong Sitting

When you are in the 21st century posture sitting, you are using muscles to balance your body. The longer you sit, the tighter the muscles get. Your body adapts to the stress.

- Overused muscles strengthen
- Underused muscles weaken
- Ligaments stretch
- Nerves may be irritated

Pain begins after the body adapts to being used in mechanically inefficient (or stressful) motions and posture patterns, causing neck and shoulder tightness, headaches, mid-back burning and low back and leg pain.

Most back pain is postural, and over time the mechanical stress causes wear and tear (i.e., arthritis/degenerative joint disease).

The Solution:

➡ **Strong Sitting Posture:**
- Push your butt back and pull your belly in to slay your slouch
- Head back and chin level
- Shoulders down and over hips
- Belly breathing

➡ **Where the toes go your nose goes**
- Keep your body facing your work.

➡ **Keep on moving**
- Move your seat's position
- Move your work's position

If the base of your chair is adjustable, tilt it forward.

If not, consider a wedge-shaped or air-filled seat pad. Be aware that using cushions and supports with a well-designed chair can remove the ergonomic benefits of the manufacturer's design.

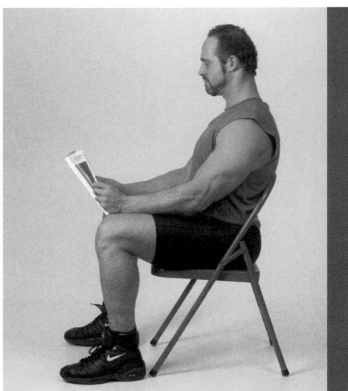
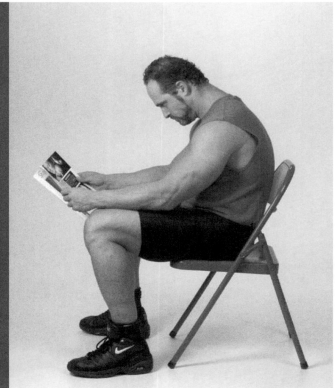
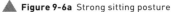

▲ **Figure 9-6a** Strong sitting posture   ▲ **Figure 9-6b** Weak sitting posture

»TRY THIS

...and standing up from sitting

When arising from a sitting position, note if your head pokes forward. If so, tuck your pelvis to stabilize your low back curves as you stand up.

Also, invest in good seating. Adjustable is good, cushioned is good in moderation (too soft= no support). And avoid low couches-they drop your hips lower than your knees, forcing your low back to round, stressing the end-range ligaments.

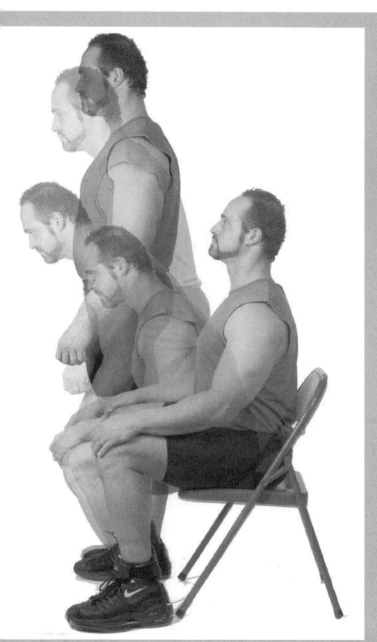

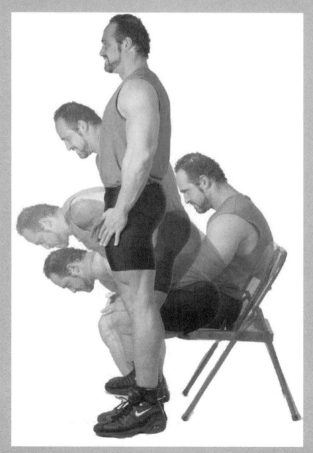

Figure 9-7a Strong standing from sitting

Figure 9-7b Weak standing from sitting

208|

»TRY THIS: *Strong Driving*

Driving

- Adjust car seat & headrest properly
    - Change seat position often during long drives or regular commutes
    - Set the rearview mirror of car a bit high to force yourself to sit with a long spine.

Driving Tucks
The first red light of the drive, sit tall and strong and do three pelvic tilts.

Getting in & out of car
- Keep your feet together and don't twist your body.
- **Getting in:**
    - Sit on the car seat
    - Do a pelvic tuck, and
    - Then pivot both feet under the wheel.
- **Getting out:**
    - Do a pelvic tuck,
    - Pivot the body, and
    - Then put both feet back on the ground, and
    - Then tuck as you stand up.

On long drives (or flights)
- Do your StrongPosture™ exercise to stretch before you start.
- Support your body occasionally.
    - There is no one perfect position...the trick is to change positions frequently.
    - Auto and plane seats usually provide weak or incorrect support. Consider back or neck pillows for your support options.
- Change positions and stretch often (the body is made to move).
    - When flying or driving try doing a sitting Angel (the arm motion of a posture angel with a pelvic tilt).
    - When driving, stop every hour or two for a few laps around the car.

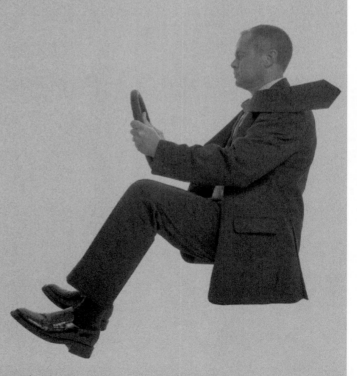

▲ **Figure 9-8** How's your driving posture?

Smart and Strong Computing

Typing is repetitive and can be really stressful. If I type sixty words per minute, that's 20,000 keystrokes per hour! When you look (or especially if you squint) at a computer screen, the head is forward of the body. Neck muscles must work to hold the head up, and back muscles must work to hold up the torso causing these muscles to become chronically tight. One solution is typing less. Another is typing differently to reduce the amount of stress on a tissue.

■ Vary your posture when typing, especially your shoulders and wrists.
■ **STRETCH** frequently to minimize the postural stress:
   ■ Do your posture exercises before and after work, and during breaks.
   ■ Do a mini-stretch of the arm and tiny muscles of the wrist every half hour during your workday.

See www.bodyzone.com/keyboardstretch to see a great keyboard wrist stretch

■ **Support your back**
   ■ Research shows decreased electrical activity of spinal muscles as well as a reduction of disc pressure with good back support.

■ **Support your arms**
   ■ Wrist, back, and neck pain can be caused by a keyboard that is too high or too low, or by resting your wrist on a sharp surface.
   ■ There is also decreased electrical activity of neck and spinal muscles when the arms are supported with an armrest.

■ **Relax your eyes**
   ■ Position your screen in front of you so you are not looking up or down.
   ■ Every so often, look at something at a distance and blink a few times.
   ■ Light right
      Eliminate glare and experiment with different lighting to find your ideal. Try soft-light halogen or full-spectrum light bulbs.

■ **Set up Smart**
   ■ Put reading materials level or close to your monitor.

■ **Choose a good chair** (and be aware the word ergonomic should mean it is bio-mechanically designed, but may also be merely marketing. Sit in it before you buy it and listen to your body).
   ■ CONSIDER SITTING ON A BALL FOR AT LEAST PART OF YOUR DAY. We do.

Relaxing

Find a good chair. Avoid an overly soft or low chairs and couches. If the hips are lower than the knees, the back rounds and pushes the spinal joints to the end of their range of motion, stressing sensitive ligaments as well as the back muscles.

210| ■   ## The Twists and Turns of Bending and Lifting

The core is your center of gravity and should be your center of motion. Tucking the pelvis slightly when beginning almost any activity "wakes up" the core so your motion patterns begin with and include these vital muscles.

Lifting

»TRY THIS: *Create a Strong Lifting LifeHabit*

Whenever you lift something
- TUCK your pelvis and pull your belly in
  - The back is stronger and more stable when the pelvis is held in a slight tuck.

- PULL back your head
- PUSH down your shoulders and then lift.

And remember

- Keep the load close to your body
  - Your center of gravity is your core, so the closer to your belly a weight is, the stronger you are.
- Bend knees, not waist
- Where the toes go the nose goes (Twist and shout, but don't twist and lift)

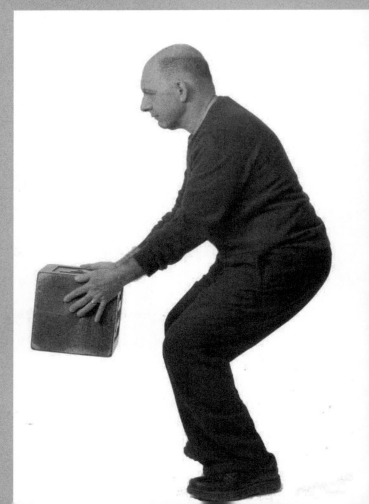

Figure 9-9 Strong lifting (belly in) vs. weak lifting (belly out)

Bending

When bending over a sink to brush your teeth, think about your stomach and notice:

> When you stand up is your stomach pulling in or pushing out?

If it is pushing out, then you are NOT using your core muscles, but the superficial back extensors.

Belly-In Lifting is pulling in your stomach to keep your nose over your toes whenever you arise from bending. For StrongPosture™ and core make a LifeHabit of crunching in your abs as the first motion you do when bending and getting up.

Loading vehicles, washing machine, mopping, vacuuming

Same story- use StrongPosture™, shifting your feet to keep load in front and close to your belly as you use your core and stand tall.

»TRY THIS

When bending over a sink to shave or put on makeup, try pulling your belly in and pressing your heels apart to stretch deep hip muscles.

Coughing and sneezing

DON'T TWIST!

- Turn so your toes and nose go the same way
- Bend your knees
- Round your back

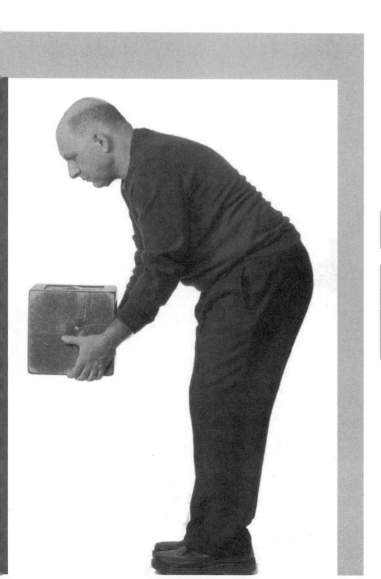

Relaxed Sleeping

Since you spend a third of you life in bed, your sleeping posture is important to get a restful night's sleep. Poor sleeping posture and support create a constant mechanical stress that can stretch muscles, ligaments, and other spinal soft tissues, leading to distortions, pain (I can't tell you how many people have come to me after "sleeping wrong" with a "crick in their back") and even long term joint damage (arthritis/DJD). Especially if you are sleep-deprived and only spend a quarter of your life in bed, you want to sleep soundly and minimize mechanical stress on the neck and spine.

What's the best bed and best pillow for me?

There are many, many beds and pillows being sold on the market...with emphasis on the word SOLD. More expensive is not necessarily better, but a cheap mattress may cost you a lot of money at the chiropractor. Be aware of marketing gimmicks (mattresses you do not have to turn over are essentially one-sided...so they may only last half as long).

If you can, always try before you buy. Sitting on the corner of a bed and bouncing up and down doesn't tell you how it feels when you are lying down. "The firmer the better" is an urban legend and not true, although if you are having an episode of acute low back pain putting a piece of plywood under your mattress may give you some temporary relief.

What's the best pillow? I like cervical pillows (the ones with two humps) of a non-rebounding material (I like memory foam). You want a pillow to be biomechanically correct for your head and neck, and it depends on how you sleep.

How should I sleep?

People sleep in one of three basic ways.
- On the side
- On the back
- On the stomach

Stomach sleeping

Change your sleeping position if you are a stomach sleeper! If you sleep on your stomach you must keep your head turned to one side to breathe, which stresses the neck and back (unless you happen to sleep on your chiropractor's table, which I do not recommend).

The body moves in a chain of motion, so spending a third of your life with your neck and spine in a stressed position causes the body to adapt to that position. Over time the neck and the supporting soft tissues will cause misalignments down the spine creating posture adaptation and distortion.

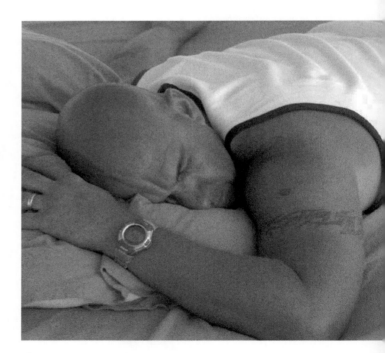

▲ **Figure 9-10** Stomach Sleeping creates neck stress

Back sleeping

Side sleeping: The best way to sleep for most of us

Sleeping on your back is good for people, especially those with a military PostureType.

■ Avoid sleeping with a thick pillow, or multiple pillows. Pushing your head forward of your body all night trains it to move that way all day.

■ A thin cervical pillow to cradle and support the neck can reduce the mechanical stress in the neck.

■ To reduce stress in the low back, try putting a pillow under the knees.

Reduce spinal stress by keeping the body aligned.

■ Keep your hips aligned with a pillow between the knees- Hips are thicker than knees, so supporting the upper leg keeps the top leg from falling in front of the body and twisting the pelvis.

■ Keep the head level with the center of the shoulders, consider a cervical pillow as thick as the distance from the side of your head to your mattress, minus how far you sink into the mattress.

■ If you aren't sure if your head is drooping down or not, ask a friend to look at you from behind when you are lying on your side. If your head is bent up or down, you are stressing the neck.

■ **Shoulder or arm problem?**
■ Support the painful arm by sleeping with that side up and a pillow between the painful arm and your body.

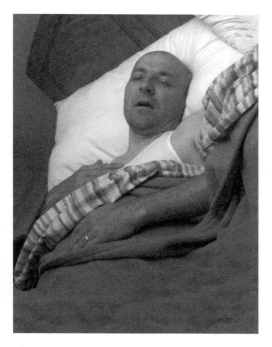

▲ **Figure 9-11** Back sleeping

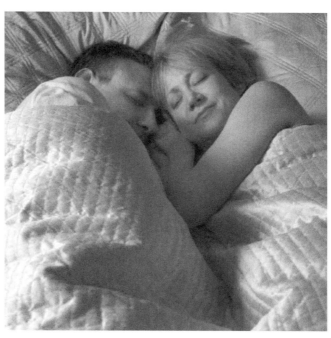

▲ **Figure 9-12** Side sleeping

Your 10 Minute a Day Program
to Keep Your Body Active and Pain-Free

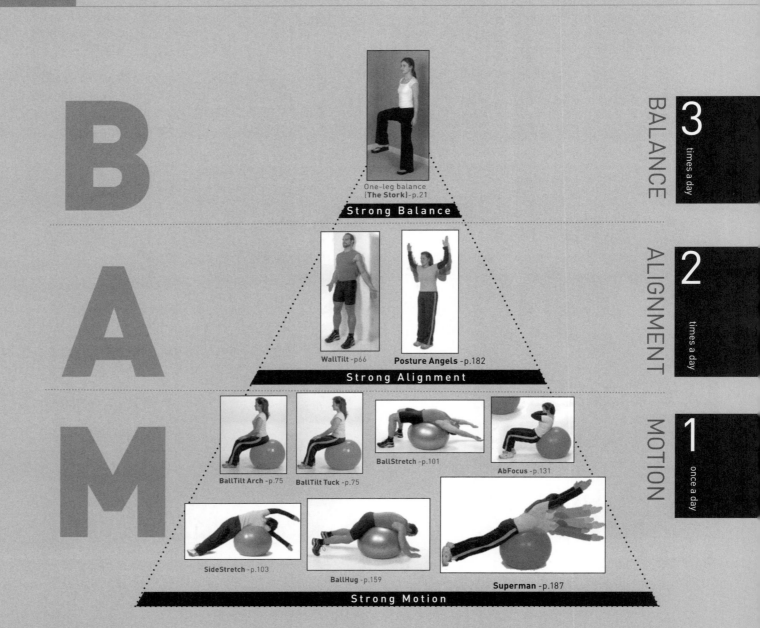

B A M

One-leg balance
[The Stork]-p.21

Strong Balance

WallTilt -p66   Posture Angels -p.182

Strong Alignment

BallTilt Arch -p.75   BallTilt Tuck -p.75

BallStretch -p.101

AbFocus -p.131

SideStretch -p.103

BallHug -p.159

Superman -p.187

Strong Motion

BALANCE   **3**   times a day

ALIGNMENT **2**   times a day

MOTION   **1**   once a day

StrongPosture™
The Path to a Lifelong Motion Cycle

Remember: *Be Posture Conscious*

Growing old does not necessarily mean feeling old. If you embrace the idea that you feel bad because you're old, so you should sit down and take it easy, then you may indeed make this become your truth. However, according to the U.S. Census, the 85-and-over age group is the fastest growing segment of our population and they are increasingly more active than at any time in history[lxxxvi]. Growing legions of older people who exercise have better balance, fewer falls, are less frail[lxxxvii, lxxxviii] and are staying active into their 80's, 90's, and beyond to prove that old doesn't necessarily equal decrepit. This trend will dramatically accelerate in the geriatric 21st century of the boomers.

From birth to death, life is a series of cycles, and posture is an omnipresent but usually unrecognized factor in many cycles, but one that we can affect. Posture shapes how your body moves, and your body's patterns of motion shape your posture in cycles both vicious and virtuous. And our sitting society, where we spend hours and hours just sitting essentially still—watching, driving, computing, and then relaxing—promotes poor posture and lack of motion.

So, if the problem is not moving, then the solution is obvious: get moving. As Nike's advertisements cry, "Just do it." Some of us do, but most people don't, as evidenced by statistics showing America getting fatter...way fatter... and more diabetic every decade. Health clubs sell three-year memberships at a fantastic discount because they know most members will not use the club after the first two weeks. Exercise classes and personal trainers help motivate

and guide, but only by consciously choosing can you create a new habit.

To change your posture, you need to teach your body a new habit. "Straighten up and don't slouch" doesn't work. In order to change how you move, you need to first become conscious of how you are moving, and then adopt new LifeHabits to consciously train new patterns of motion and so retrain the body to move unconsciously in those new patterns of motion.

You have to use it or lose it

In other words

Use it to keep it

So even though there is no one perfect posture, strengthening your posture with daily posture exercises as part of your regular physical activity will help you keep moving well as you age. In other words, stand taller today to live longer tomorrow!

APPENDIX **A**

Sample 7 week Stand Taller~Live Longer posture exercise progression.

Along with one-leg standing Balance exercises, integrating the wall protocol for strong Alignment and the ball protocol for strong Motion can form the backbone of a daily posture exercise program. The following summary of the exercises in this book is for educational purposes only. Consult your physician, doctor of chiropractic, trainer or Certified Posture Exercise Professional (CPEP) for advice and modifications for your specific clinical and bio-mechanical goals and considerations.

Strong Balance: *3 times a day*
Strong Alignment: *2 times a day*
Strong Motion: *1 time a day.*

Week 1
Strong Balance: *One-Leg Balance*
Strong Alignment: *BallSit*

Week 2
Strong Balance: *One-Leg Balance*
Strong Alignment: *BallSit BallMarch*
Strong Motion: *5 Breaths*

Week 3
Strong Balance: *One-Leg Balance*
Strong Alignment: *WallTilt, BallSit*
Strong Motion: *BallTilt*

Week 4
Strong Balance: *One-Leg Balance*
Strong Alignment: *WallTilt*
Strong Motion: *BallTilt > BallStretch > SideStretch*

Week 5
Strong Balance: *One-Leg Balance*
Strong Alignment: *WallTilt > Neck Retractions > SeeSaw*
Strong Motion: *BallTilt > BackStretch > AbFocus > SideStretch*

Week 6
Strong Balance: *One-Leg Balance*
Strong Alignment: *WallTilt > ArmsUP*
Strong Motion: *BallTilt > BackStretch > AbFocus > SideStretch > BallHug*

Week 7
Strong Balance: *One-Leg Balance*
Strong Alignment: *Posture Angels*
Strong Motion: *BallTilt > BackStretch > AbFocus > Sidestretch > BallHug > Superman*

APPENDIX B

Q: What do I do if it hurts?

Realistically, sometimes things may hurt, but there are natural solutions to many of life's pains. I'm a big fan of cold packs, hot baths, topicals, massage, and some neutraceuticals such as glucosamine, MSM, and chondroitin.

Do I use Hot or Cold for drug-free pain control?

A: Cold reduces circulation
Heat increases circulation

So, if it's a new injury cold is the best bet for minimizing swelling, at least for the first two or three days. Swelling can cause as much tissue damage as the original injury, and can be prevented with fifteen minutes of ice compression, three times a day, to reduce pain and promote healing. Flexible gelpacks are easier to use than ice cubes in a plastic bag, or a bag of frozen peas. Be sure to use a towel to protect your skin.

Moist heat can be good for sore and tight muscles, but severe spasms may also respond better to cold initially. For joint injuries try alternating hot and cold compresses after the first three days, although many people will still find that while heat feels better while it is on, ice makes it feel better later on.

For more self-help ideas to control acute and chronic back pain, see www.bodyzone.com/backpainselfhelp. If pain persists, consult a professional.

TABLE OF **IMAGES**

REFERENCES

i- WSJ 10/21/03 According to the Federal Highway Administration, the time the average American spends behind the wheel: 1990: 49 minutes / day2001: 62.5 minutes / day , extra 80 hrs a year.

ii- "Chronic back pain, often with associated leg pain, is the most common medical complaint in developed countries, (Bigos, et al., 1994). Headache is its only peer, (Lawrence, 1977). Costs associated with back pain are enormous, (Kelsey, 1982)." From Textbook of Pain, 4th Edition, 1999, "Chronic Back Pain," Donlin M. Long, USA:Introduction.

iii- Half of all computer workers suffer pain (Neck and shoulder 67%; LBP 40%; Wrist pain 29%) US Dept of Labor, 1991.

iv- Height Loss in Older Men- Associations with Total Mortality and Incidence of Cardiovascular Disease. S. Goya Wannamethee, PhD; A. Gerald Shaper, FRCP; Lucy Lennon, MSc; Peter H. Whincup, FRCP, PhD, Arch Intern Med. 2006; 166:2546-2552.

v - Low Back Disorders, Stuart McGill, 2002 Kinetic Press.

vi- Harvard Medical School Adviser, Harvard Publishing, January 24, 2006.

vii- Stronger back muscles reduce the incidence of vertebral fractures: a prospective 10-year follow-up of postmenopausal women. Sinaki M, Itoi E, Wahner HW, Wollan P, Gelzcer R, Mullan BP, Collins DA, Hodgson SF. Department of Physical Medicine and Rehabilitation, Mayo Clinic, Rochester, MN 55905, USA.
The long-term protective effect of stronger back muscles on the spine was determined in 50 healthy white postmenopausal women, aged 58-75 years, 8 years after they had completed a 2-year randomized, controlled trial. Twenty-seven subjects had performed progressive, resistive back-strengthening exercises for 2 years and 23 had served as controls. Bone mineral density, spine radiographs, back extensor strength, biochemical marker values, and level of physical activity were obtained for all subjects at baseline, 2 years, and 10 years. Mean back extensor strength (BES) in the back-exercise (BE) group was 39.4 kg at baseline, 66.8 kg at 2 years (after 2 years of prescribed exercises), and 32.9 kg at 10 years (8 years after cessation of the prescribed exercises). Mean BES in the control (C) group was 36.9 kg at baseline, 49.0 kg at 2 years, and 26.9 kg at 10 years. The difference between the two groups was still statistically significant at 10-year follow-up (p = 0.001). The difference in bone mineral density, which was not significant between the two groups at baseline and 2-year follow-up, was significant at 10-year follow-up (p =

0.0004). The incidence of vertebral compression fracture was 14 fractures in 322 vertebral bodies examined (4.3%) in the C group and 6 fractures in 378 vertebral bodies examined (1.6%) in the BE group (chi-square test, p = 0.0290). The relative risk for compression fracture was 2.7 times greater in the C group than in the BE group. To our knowledge, this is the first study reported in the literature demonstrating the long-term effect of strong back muscles on the reduction of vertebral fractures in estrogen-deficient women.

viii- Reducing the risk of falls through proprioceptive dynamic posture training in osteoporotic women with kyphotic posturing: a randomized pilot study. Sinaki M, Lynn SG. Department of Physical Medicine and Rehabilitation, Mayo Clinic, Rochester, Minnesota, USA. Am J Phys Med Rehabil. 2002, Apr 81(4):241-6.
OBJECTIVE: To assess the effect of a proprioceptive dynamic posture training program on balance in osteoporotic women with kyphotic posture. DESIGN: Subjects were randomly assigned to either a proprioceptive dynamic posture training program or exercise only group. Anthropometric measurements, muscle strength, level of physical activity, computerized dynamic posturography, and spine radiography were performed at baseline and 1 mo. RESULTS: At the 1-mo follow-up, three groups were formed on the basis of the baseline computerized dynamic posturography results. In general, groups 1 and 2 had no significant change at 1 mo, whereas group 3 improved balance significantly at 1 mo. CONCLUSION: The subjects who had abnormal balance and used the proprioceptive dynamic posture training program had the most significant improvement in balance. Improved balance could reduce the risk of falls.

ix- Musculoskeletal conditions, including arthritis, low back pain and repetitive motion strain, are the leading cause of absenteeism. Institute for Health and Productivity Management (IHPM), 2002.

x- 60% of U.S. adults reported back pain. 83% of Americans rely on OTC pain relievers. 2/3 of the people with back pain in the past can expect some symptoms every year. 2/3 of Americans expect life stresses & pressures to increase their pain.1/5 had physical pain during at least 20 days of last month. 40% of employed said lifting and carrying cause significant pain. Commuting to and from work, and/or driving long distances, are significant sources of pain. ORUDIS(R) KT(TM) Pain Relief 2000, Pain in the 1990s, the Increasing Prevalence of Pain in the Lives of Americans. Yankelovich Partners, an opinion research firm.

xi- "Lower back pain is one of the most common reasons for medical visits. Two of every three people have suffered from lower back pain at some time in their lives; the annual incidence is 2 percent to 5 percent." Kelley's Textbook of Internal Medicine, Fourth Edition, 2000, "Approach to the Patient with Back Pain," written by Glen S. O'Sullivan, U.S.A.

xii- Basics in Geriatrics, the Emory Big 10. Joseph Ouslander, MD, Metro Atlanta MD news, November/December 2002.

xiii- Gait variability and fall risk in community-living older adults: a 1-year prospective study. Hausdorff, JM; Rios, DA; Edelber, HK. Archives of Physical Medicine and Rehabilitation 2001; 82(8):1050–6.

xiv- Centers for Disease Control and Prevention, National Center for Injury Prevention and Control. Web-based Injury Statistics Query and Reporting System (WISQARS) (cited 2006 Oct 9). Available from URL: www.cdc.gov/ncipc/wisqars.

xv- Changes in the Cross-sectional Area of Multifidus and Psoas in Patients with Unilateral Back Pain: the Relationship to Pain and Disability. Barker, Karen L. PhD, MCSP*; Shamley, Delva R. PhD; Jackson, David PhD, MCSP. Spine. 29(22):E515-E519, November 15, 2004.

xvi- Aging alone does not generally cause pain. Geriatric syndromes (i.e., gait instability) are commonly undiagnosed and therefore not managed optimally. Small changes in functional capability (e.g., the ability to transfer) can make a critical difference for quality of life of older patients. Core strength and control is what makes the difference being able to do, or not. Basics in Geriatrics, Joseph Ouslander, MD, Metro Atlanta MD news, November/December 2002.

xvii- Hyperkyphotic Posture Predicts Mortality in Older Community-Dwelling Men and Women: A Prospective Study. Deborah M. Kado, MD, MS*, Mei-Hua Huang, DrPH*, Arun S. Karlamangla, MD, PhD*, Elizabeth Barrett-Connor, MD and Gail A. Greendale, MD*, Journal of the American Geriatrics Society, volume 52, issue 10, Page 1662, October 2004, doi:10.1111/j.1532-5415.2004.52458.x

xviii- Usefulness of posture training for patients with temporomandibular disorders, Edward f. Wright, D.D.S., M.S., Manuel A. Domenech, PH.D. and Joseph R. Fischer Jr., M.S. J Am Dent Assoc, volume 131, no 2, 202-210.

xix- Single leg stand test from Shirley A. Sahrmann: Diagnosis and Treatment of Movement Impairment Syndromes; Publ. Mosby 2002.

xx- The ability to balance on one leg for five seconds can predict which elderly people are most at risk for injury from a fall. 3 year study of 300 community-living persons over 60. 70% of these healthy older persons had at least one fall. Subjects who were unable to balance on one leg had 2.1 times the risk injury from a fall. No link between the number of medications the elderly people were on at the beginning of the trial and their risk for falling. The risk for an injurious fall increases with age. CONCLUSION: One-leg standing balance could "reasonably" identify those with a greater risk of injurious falls and who are possibly more likely to benefit from an intervention trial. Dr. Bruno J. Vellas, Journal of the American Geriatrics Society, 1997; 45:735-738.

xxi- Dynamic stabilization training requires some cortical (or conscious) effort, but once it is trained, a new motor program will form that will sub cortically (unconsciously) protect vulnerable joints from injury on a reflex, semi- automatic basis. To facilitate the formation of a new motor program, labile surfaces (i.e. PostureBalls)...challenge balance so afferent pathways are spontaneously facilitated in a concentrated way. Liebenson C, DC. Dynamic Chiropractic, 1998; 16(20):36, 40, 41.

xxii- The effects of a wobble board exercise training program on static balance performance and strength of lower extremity muscles. Balogun JA, Adesinasi CO, Marzouk DK. Physiotherapy CAN 1992; 44:23-30.

xxiii- Clinical Biomechanics of the spine, Punjabi and White; Lippincott, Williams and Wilkins, 1990.

xxiv- "Stability: From a biomechanical concept to chiropractic practice," Stuart McGill, Canadian Chiropractic Journal, 1999/ 43/2, with permission.

xxv- ibid

xxvi- Outer Unit Obliques Posterior Oblique system: Lats to contra lateral Gmax. Anterior Oblique: Internal and external abdominal obliques to contralateral thigh adductors
Deep Longitudinal System: Compresses the SI joint- ES to thoraco-dorsal fascia to contralateral sacrotuberous ligament and biceps femoris
Lateral System: Glut med, Glut min, and contralateral thigh adductors

xxvii- On a segmental spinal level, the co-contraction, or co-activation of the deep spinal muscles, especially the multifidus, with the deep abdominal muscles, especially the TrA, provides the "corset" to stabilize the mobile spine, preventing ligamentous injury. The multifidus is weak in most acute LBP and atrophied on MRI's of patients with a history of low back problems, even in

the absence of active symptoms. "Multifidus Muscle Recovery in Acute Low Back Pain Patients." Hides JA.
University of Queensland, 1996.

xxviii- I Fast twitch muscle fibers: work hard, contract with strong force for a short period of time. Postural
II Slow twitch muscle fibers: can't work as hard, but have much greater endurance. Phasic. Muscles shake

Type I POSTURAL MUSCLE CHARACTERISTICS	Type II POSTURAL MUSCLE CHARACTERISTICS
Anti-gravity & tonic Higher resting tonus than phasic muscles	Are available on demand but do not oppose gravity
Tend toward shortness and tightness	Tend toward inhibition and weakness
Less reactive to injury	More reactive to injury
Atrophy less quickly than phasic muscles	Atrophy more quickly than postural muscles

xxix- The control of standing is a complicated task that involves the action of muscles distributed over the whole body. Forces arising from gravity, external events or our own actions all tend to disturb the unstable equilibrium that preserves posture. For the central nervous system the problem of standing can be cast in terms of finding appropriate relations among body segments to maintain the desired position of the body as a whole with respect to the environment.
The control of upright stance involves predictable and unpredictable perturbations in the interplay of perceptual information, attention and cognitive processes in the control of standing.
Ramesh Balasubramaniam and Alan M. Wing,
Trends in Cognitive Sciences, 2002, 6:12:531-536

xxx- The two main functions of the postural control system
Resist gravity and maintain balance
Fix the orientation and position of the segments that serve as a reference frame for perception and action with respect to the external world.

This dual function of postural control is based on four components:
Reference values, such as orientation of body segments and position of the center of gravity (an internal representation of the body or postural body scheme)
Multisensory inputs regulating orientation and stabilization of body segments
Postural stabilization and balance recovery during voluntary movement.
Jean Massion, Current Opinion in Neurobiology 1994, 4:877-887.

xxxi- Three-dimensional motion patterns during active bending in patients with chronic low back pain. Lund T, Nydegger T, Schlenzka D, Oxland TR. Spine 2002 Sep 1;27(17):1865-74.

xxxii- Impaired postural control of the lumbar spine is associated with delayed muscle response times in Pts w CLBP. Radebold, MD et al. Spine 2001;26:724-30.

xxxiii- Korr, PhD. JAOA 1991;91(2): 156,161-8, 170.

xxxiv- Three-dimensional motion patterns during active bending in patients with chronic low back pain. Lund T, Nydegger T, Schlenzka D, Oxland TR. Spine 2002 Sep 1;27(17):1865-74.

xxxv- Evaluation of specific stabilizing exercise in the treatment of chronic low back pain with radiologic diagnosis of spondylolysis or spondylolysthesis. O'Sullivan P, Twomey L, Allison G 1997. Spine 24:2959-2967.

xxxvi- Exercise for low back pains should incorporate a controlled contraction of the transverse abdominus (TrA) independently of the global muscles. Independent of other abdominal muscles, contracting the TrA significantly decreased the laxity of the SIJ to a larger extant than a bracing action using the rest of the lateral abdominal muscles. "The relation between the TrA, SIJ mechanics, and LBP," Richards, Snijders, Hides. Spine 2002:27(4) 399-406.

xxxvii- "Proposed Mechanism for Chronic Back Pain," MM Panjabi. European Spine Journal, July 27, 2005:
A hypothesis of chronic back pain: How Ligament subfailure injuries lead to muscle control dysfunction
Injured Tissues that Contain Mechanoreceptors(From Either Single Macrotrauma or Repeated Microtrauma)
~Altered Ligamentous Mechanical Neurological Afferent Input
Into the Central Nervous System ("Corrupted Transducer Signals")

-Altered Spinal Neuromuscular Unit Control

-Altered Motor Output to the Muscles ("Corrupted Muscle Response Pattern")

-Altered Coordination of Individual Muscle Activation

-Altered Muscular Mechanical Neurological Afferent Input into The Central Nervous System

(More "Corrupted Transducer Signals")

-Higher Mechanical Loading to the Facet Joints

-Increased Muscle Fatigue

-Higher Stresses and Strains in Ligaments, Muscles, and Mechanoreceptors

- "Adverse Consequences"

- "Tissue Inflammation"

-Acceleration of Disc and Facet Degeneration

-"Chronic Back Pain"

xxxviii- "Low back injury is ...(from...)...a history of excessive loading which gradually, but progressively, reduces the tissue failure tolerance." McGill SM 1998. Low back exercises: prescription for the healthy back and when recovering from injury. In: Resources Manual for Guidelines for Exercise Testing and Prescription. 3rd ed. Indianapolis, IN: American College of Sports Medicine. Baltimore, Williams and Wilkins.

xxxiv- NIOSH Publican No. 97-141: Musculoskeletal Disorders and Workplace Factors: Critical Review of Epidemiologic Evidence for Work-Related Musculoskeletal Disorders of the Neck, Upper Extremity, and Low Back, July 1997. http://www.cdc.gov/niosh/docs/97-141/ergoref.html.

xl- "Are individuals with back pain at heightened risk of permanent spinal injury?" Wiesel, S, MD. Backletter 2002;17(1): 1, 8-10.

xli- CDC study found per Reuters http://www.msnbc.msn.com/id/15734242/).

xlii- Inflammation and pain result in voluntary inhibition of muscle activity across the affected joint. "Immobilization or early mobilization after an acute soft tissue injury?" Kannus, MD, PhD. Phys & Sportsmed 2000; 28(3): 55-63.

xliii- A. Vania Apkarian, The Journal of Neuroscience. Nov. 23, 2004.

xliv- "A Reassessment of Normal Cervical Range of Motion," Skip Lantz, Jiri Dvorak, MD, et al, Spine, June 15, 2003.

xlv- "The effects of failure feedback and pain-related fear on pain report, pain tolerance, and pain avoidance in chronic low back pain patients." Van den Hout JHC, Vlaeyen JWS, Houben RMA, Soeters APM, Peters ML. Pain 2001;92:247-257.

xlvi- "Just N. Pain expectancy and work disability in patients with acute and chronic pain: A test of the fear avoidance hypothesis." Ciccione DS, Journal of Pain 2001;2:181-194.

xlvii- "A systematic review of psychological factors as predictors of chronicity/disability in prospective cohorts of low back pain," Pincus T, Burton A, Vogel S, Field AP. Spine 2002;27:E109-120.

xlviii- "The stabilizing system of the spine. Part 1. Function, dysfunction, adaptation, and enhancement," Panjabi MM. J Spinal Disorders 1992;5:383-389.

xlix- "Creep response of the lumbar spine to prolonged full flexion" McGill SM, Brown S. Clin Biomech 1992;7:43-46.

l- Donatelli, Orthopedic Physical Therapy, 2nd ed, NY Churchill Livingston, 1994, 1-31.

li- If a soft tissue injury is not completely healed within 6 weeks, there is probably poor blood supply of uncontrolled mechanical stresses exceeding the tolerance of the healing tissues. Tissues which fail to heal over 6 to 8 wks probably will not heal itself & should be considered a chronic injury. Mooney, MD. J Musculoskeletal Med 1995; Oct: 33-39.

lii- The majority of injuries to the low back involve soft tissues or discs such as sprains and strains of musculo ligamentous tissues, which have a relatively brief healing period. When healing is temporally complete, but biomechanically imperfect, it leads to permanent impairment of supporting elements, and chronic disability may follow. Mayer TG, MD. Neurologic Clinics/North America 1999;17(1):131-147.

liii- Repetitive noxious stimulation of unmyelinated C-fibers can result in prolonged discharge of dorsal horn cells. This phenomenon which is termed "wind-up", is a progressive increase in the number of action potentials elicited per stimulus that occurs in dorsal horn neurons.36 Repetitive episodes of "wind-up" may precipitate long-term potentiation (LTP), which involves a long lasting increase in the efficacy of synaptic transmission. Where "wind-up" is thought to last only minutes, LTP by definition, lasts at least one hour and maybe even months. Both "wind–up" and LTP are believed to be part of the sensitization process involved in many chronic pain states.

Animal studies suggest that expansion of receptive fields may also occur following tissue injury. Therefore, any peripheral stimulation would activate a greater number of dorsal horn cells because of an increased overlap of their receptive fields.

Evidence suggests that excessive nociceptive input to the dorsal horn can have excitotoxic consequences resulting in the death of inhibitory interneurons. This inhibition may contribute to spinal hyper–excitability.

The allodynia and hyperalgesia associated with neuropathic pain may be best explained by: 1) the development of spontaneous activity of afferent input 2) the sprouting of large primary efferents (eg. A–beta fibers from lamina 3 into lamina 1 and 2), 3) sprouting of sympathetic efferents into neuromas and dorsal root and ganglion cells, 4) elimination of intrinsic modulatory systems and 5) up regulation of receptors in the dorsal horn which mediate excitatory processes.

Understanding Neuropathic Pain, Steven Richeimer MD. FOR MORE INFO SEE

http://www.spineuniverse.com/displayarticle.php/article1614.html.

liv- "Spontaneous Pain, Both Neuropathic and Inflammatory, Is Related to Frequency of Spontaneous Firing in Intact C-Fiber Nociceptors," Laiche Djouhri, Stella Koutsikou, Xin Fang, Simon McMullan, and Sally N. Lawson, Department of Physiology, Medical School, University of Bristol, Bristol BS8 1TD, United Kingdom, The Journal of Neuroscience, January 25, 2006, 26(4):1281-1292; doi:10.1523/JNEUROSCI.3388-05.2006.

lv- Waddell G. MD. The Back Pain Revolution. Churchill Livingstone 1998: 151-151.

lvi- Giacomo Rizzolatti, Leonardo Fogassi and Vittorio Gallese, Mirrors in the Mind, Scientific American, November 2006.

lvii- Vilayanur S. Ramachandran and Lindsay M. Oberman, Broken Mirrors: A Theory of Autism, Scientific American, November 2006.

lviii- Leon Chaitow N.D., D.O., M.R.O., Osteopathy: A Complete Health Care System, Leon Chaitow N.D., D.O., M.R.O., from The Principles of Osteopathy http://www.healthy.net/scr/article.asp?Id=1876.

lix- Selye, Hans, The Stress of Life, New York, McGraw, 1956.

lx- "Change of Complexity Patterns in Human Posture during Aging," Stefan Thurnera,b, Christian Mittermaierc, Klaus Ehrenbergera. Department of Otorhinolaryngology, Institute of Mathematics, andDepartment of Physical Medicine, University of Vienna, Audiology & Neuro-Otology 2002;7:240-248 (DOI: 10.1159/000063740).

lxi- Fleck SJ, Kraemer WJ. Designing Resistance Training Programs. Champaign, IL: Human Kinetics, 1987.

lxii- "Archive of Soft Tissue Injuries, a review of the literature," Kelet, J. Med Science Sports Exercise, 1986, 18(5)489-50.

lxiii- Background: Massage therapy is an attractive treatment option for osteoarthritis (OA), but its efficacy is uncertain. We conducted a randomized, controlled trial of massage therapy for OA of the knee.
Methods: Sixty-eight adults with radiographically confirmed OA of the knee were assigned either to treatment (twice-weekly sessions of standard Swedish massage in weeks 1-4 and once-weekly sessions in weeks 5-8) or to control (delayed intervention). Primary outcomes were changes in the Western Ontario and McMaster Universities Osteoarthritis Index (WOMAC) pain and functional scores and the visual analog scale of pain assessment. The sample provided 80% statistical power to detect a 20-point difference between groups in the change from baseline on the WOMAC and visual analog scale, with a 2-tailed of .05.

Results: The group receiving massage therapy demonstrated significant improvements in the mean (SD) WOMAC global scores (–17.44 [23.61] mm; P<.001), pain (–18.36 [23.28]; P<.001), stiffness (–16.63 [28.82] mm; P<.001), and physical function domains (–17.27 [24.36] mm; P <.001) and in the visual analog scale of pain assessment (–19.38 [28.16] mm; P<.001), range of motion in degrees (3.57 [13.61]; P = .03), and time to walk 50 ft (15 m) in seconds (–1.77 [2.73]; P<.01). Findings were unchanged in multivariable models controlling for demographic factors.

Conclusions: Massage therapy seems to be efficacious in the treatment of OA of the knee. Further study of cost effectiveness and duration of treatment effect is clearly warranted.
"Massage Therapy for Osteoarthritis of the Knee: A Randomized Controlled Trial," Perlman AI, et al. Archives of Internal Medicine. December 11/25, 2007; Vol. 166; No. 22, pp. 2533-2538.

lxiv- from wikipedia
The Hubel and Wiesel experiments greatly expanded the scientific knowledge of sensory processing. In one experiment, done in 1959, they inserted a microelectrode into the primary visual cortex of an anesthetized cat. They then projected patterns of light and dark on a screen in front of the cat. They found that some neurons fired rapidly when presented with lines at one angle, while others responded best to another angle. Some of these neurons responded differently to light patterns than to dark patterns. Hubel and Wiesel called these neurons "simple cells." Still other neurons, which they termed "complex cells," had identical responses to light and dark patterns. These studies showed how the visual system constructs complex representations of visual information from simple stimulus features (Goldstein, 2001).

Hubel and Wiesel received the Nobel Prize for two major contributions: 1. their work on development of the visual system, which involved a description of ocular dominance columns in the 1960s and 1970s; and 2. their work establishing a foundation for visual neurophysiology, describing how signals from the eye are processed by the brain to generate edge detectors, motion detectors, stereoscopic depth detectors and color detectors, building blocks of the visual scene. By depriving kittens from using one eye, they showed that columns in the primary visual cortex receiving inputs from the other eye took over the areas that would normally receive input from the deprived eye. This has important implications for the understanding of deprivation amblyopia, a type of visual loss due to unilateral visual deprivation during the so-called "critical period". These kittens also did not develop areas receiving input from both eyes, a feature needed for binocular vision. Hubel and Wiesel's experiments showed that the ocular dominance develops irreversibly early in childhood development. These studies opened the door for the understanding and treatment of childhood cataracts and strabismus. They were also important in the study of cortical plasticity (Goldstein, 2001).

lxv- Thomas Hanna, Body Somatics, 1990, Da Capo Press ,ISBN-10: 0201079798,ISBN-13: 978-0201079791.

lxvi- Contemporary terminology for models of cellular learning and memory.
Use-dependent change in synaptic strength,
Synaptic plasticity,
Synaptic long-term plasticity in nociceptive systems,
Use-dependent long term potentiation of synaptic strength
Injury induced hyperalgesia"Learning and memory in pain pathways," Sandkuhler J. Pain 2000;88:113-118. "Patterns of Motion & Pain," Gerontology 2001 Jul-Aug;47(4):189-94.

lxvii- Animals' blindness was due to a complex molecular process called long-term depression. That process, which scientists have studied for years, occurs when the connections between neurons get the wrong signals, making them weaker and liable to die. A molecule called glutamate acts as a messenger that lets neurons communicate. For a neuron to receive a message, it must have a glutamate receptor. In long-term depression, which is prompted by the wrong type of input, those receptors are modified and removed, leading connections, or synapses, to wither away.
"Molecular mechanism for loss of visual cortical responsiveness following brief monocular deprivation," Heynen, A.J., Yoon, B.-J., Liu, C.-H., Chung, H.J., Huganir, R.L. and Bear, M.F. Nature Neuroscience, 2003 6(8): 854-86.

lxviii-
http://www.boston.com/globe/search/stories/reprints/finallythe072903.htm

lxix- Injury damaged proprioceptors show localized proprioceptive loss in the trunk muscles & ligaments and resulting in low back pain. "Impaired Postural Control of the Lumbar Spine Is Associated With Delayed Muscle Response Times in Patients With Chronic Idiopathic Low Back Pain," Radebold, Andrea MD; Cholewicki, Jacek PhD; Polzhofer, Gert K. BA; Greene, Hunter S. MD. Spine. 26(7):724-730, April 1, 2001.

lxx- "Power Training Improves Balance in Healthy Older Adults," Rhonda Orr1,, Nathan J. de Vos1, Nalin A. Singh2,3, Dale A. Ross3, Theodora M. Stavrinos3 and Maria A. Fiatarone-Singh1,4,5. The Journals of Gerontology Series A: Biological Sciences and Medical Sciences 61:78-85 (2006).

lxxi- "Inefficient muscular stabilization of the lumbar spine associated with low back pain," 10. Hodges PW, Richardson CA. Spine 1996; 21:2640-2650.

lxxii- "Delayed postural contraction of the transverse abdominus associated with movement of the lower limb in people with low back pain," Hodges PW, Richardson CA. J Spinal Disord 1998; 11:46-56.

lxxiii- "Evidence of lumbar multifidus muscle-wasting ipsilateral to symptoms in patients with acute/subacute low back pain," Hides JA, Stokes MJ, Saide M, Jull Ga, Cooper DH. Spine 1993; 19(2):165-172.

lxiv- McGill SM, 2000. Clinical biomechanics of the thoracolumbar spine in Clinical Biomechanics (ed Dvir Z),

lxxv- Resistance exercises for trunk extension can be performed with symmetry or asymmetry of extensor musculature. Symmetry of motion is usually seen in patients without back problems, and asymmetry is typical of people with back problems. "Decoupling of bilateral paraspinal excitation in subjects with low back pain,"
Grabiner MD, Koh TJ, Ghazawi AE. Spine 1992; 17:1219.

lxxvi- "Multifidus muscle recovery is not automatic after resolution of acute, first-episode of low back pain," Hides JA, Richardson CA, Jull GA. Spine 1996a; 21(23):2763-2769.

lxxvii- "Mulitifidus muscle rehabilitation decreases recurrence of symptoms following first episode of low back pain," Hides JA, Richardson CA, Jull GA. Proceedings of the National Congress of the Australian Physiotherapy Association, Brisbane, per Liebensehn, Mechanism of Injury of the Spine, Dynamic Chiropractic 11/30/2000, http://findarticles.com/p/articles/mi_qa3987/is_200011/ai_n8923706.

lxxviii- "Neuromuscular trunk performance and spinal loading during a fatiguing isometric trunk extension with varying torque requirements," Sparto PJ, Paarnianpour M, Massa WS, Granata KP, Reinsel TE, Simon S. Spine 1997; 10:145-156.

lxxix- "Static back endurance and the risk of low-back pain," Luuto S, Heliovaara M, Hurri H, Alaranta H. Clin Biomech 1995; 10:323-324.

lxxx- "Physical measurements as risk indicators for low-back trouble over a one-year period," Biering-Sorensen F. Spine 1984; 9:106-119.

lxxxi- Arthritis and Rheumatism, 1997, James F. Fries, M.D. and associates described their data, which studied 410 members of a runners club and 289 community control subjects over a 6 year period. The average age of the men and women in the study was 60 to 66 years.
The data from this study indicate a lower degree of pains in the muscles and joints in those subjects who ran regularly compared to those who did not run. This effect of running was particularly significant in women. The study found that runners not only had decreased mortality, but also had significantly less disability than non-runners.

lxxxii- Running and Joint Issues, Wall Street Journal, June 8, 2004.

lxxxiii- The effect of running on the pathogenesis of osteoarthritis of the hips and knees. vClin Orthop 1985 Sep;(198):106-9.

lxxxiv- American College of Sports Medicine http://www.acsm.org/Content/NavigationMenu/Research/Roundtables_Specialty_Conf/PastRoundtables/Exercise_for_Older_Adults.htm

lxxxv- "Exercise type and intensity in relation to coronary heart disease in men," Tanasescu M, Leitzmann MF, et al. Journal of the American Medical Association 2002:288(16), pp. 1994-2000.

lxxxvi- www.census.gov

lxxxvii- Exercise can help balance # Judge, J. O., Lindsey, C., Underwood, M., and D. WINSEMIUS. Balance improvements in older women: effects of exercise training. Phys. Ther. 73:254-265, 1993.

lxxxviii- Wolf, S. L., H. X. Barnhart, N. G. Kutner, E. McNeely, C. Coogler, and T. XU. Reducing frailty and falls in older persons: an investigation of Tai Chi and computerized balance training--Atlanta FICSIT Group: Frailty and Injuries--Cooperative Studies of Intervention Techniques. J. Am. Geriatr. Soc. 44:489-497, 1996. [see "xci"]

TABLE OF ONLINE **LINKS**

Muscle anatomy information- www.bodyzone.com\
muscleanatomy.

Brain, nerves and control system anatomy and information-
www.bodyzone.com/braincontrol

Core information- www.bodyzone.com/coremuscleinfo

Kegel Exercises and strengthening the pelvic floor -
www.bodyzone.com/kegel

Patterns of motion- www.bodyzone.com/Patterns

Isometric vs isokinetic exercise- www.strongposture.com/
isokinetic

Computer keyboard wrist stretch-
www.bodyzone.com/keyboardstretch

Self-help for acute and chronic back pain (If pain persists,
consult a professional) -
www.bodyzone.com/backpainselfhelp

TABLE OF ONLINE **RESOURCES**

For more StrongPosture™ information, visit
www.standtallerlivelonger.com

Online and local vendors for StrongPosture™ tools &
advice: www.BodyZone.com/resources

For Balls, Foam Rollers, Exercise Tubing and other tools
for Posture Practices: www.PostureZone.com

Find a Certified Posture Exercise Professional (CPEP) near
you who teaches StrongPosture™ exercises:
www.bodyzone.com/CPEPs

Find a doctor or chiropractic near you, visit
www.bodyzone.com/chiropractic
Find a massage therapist near you, visit
www.bodyzone.com/massage

230|

ABOUT THE **AUTHOR**

Since graduating from New York Chiropractic College, Dr. Steven Weiniger has focused on posture rehabilitation and biomechanics in private clinical practice outside of Atlanta, Georgia. In addition to caring for patients, Dr. Weiniger serves as Managing Partner of BodyZone.com, an online educational resource for professionals and the general public.

As a post graduate instructor, he lectures nationally on posture and the importance of integrating exercise into every lifestyle. Through his seminars, Integrating Chiropractic & Posture Rehab Exercise, and Clinical Posture Assessment, Therapy & Exercise, Dr. Weiniger has trained thousands of doctors and other health professionals in his StrongPosture™ protocols for rehab care and keeping patients moving well as they age.

He authored the Posture Assessment chapter in the Photographic Manual of Regional Orthopedic and Neurological Tests, and his articles on posture, anti-aging, exercise, and practice management are published by newspapers and journals across the country.

Dr. Weiniger has served as a board director for multiple professional health care organizations. In 2005, Dr. Weiniger was an appointed delegate to the White House Conference on Aging (WHCoA), a once a decade event to develop recommendations for the President and Congress on issues, policy and research in the field of aging. He later shared his expertise and findings at the National Chiropractic Legislative Conference (NCLC).

Dr. Weiniger enjoys recumbent cycling, skiing, and yoga, and resides in Roswell, Georgia with his wife and family.

INDEX